Life in the Asperger Lane

Dan Coulter's Collected

Asperger Articles

Volume 1

By Dan Coulter

coultervideo publishing

(A division of Coulter Video, Inc.)
1428 Pinecroft Drive
Winston-Salem, NC 27104

Cover Design by Julie Coulter

Life in the Asperger Lane
All Rights Reserved.
No part of this book may be used or reproduced
in any manner whatsoever without the written permission of the author.
www.coultervideo.com

Copyright © 2012 Dan Coulter

All rights reserved.

ISBN: 0615630766
ISBN-13: 978-0615630762

This book is dedicated to Drew.

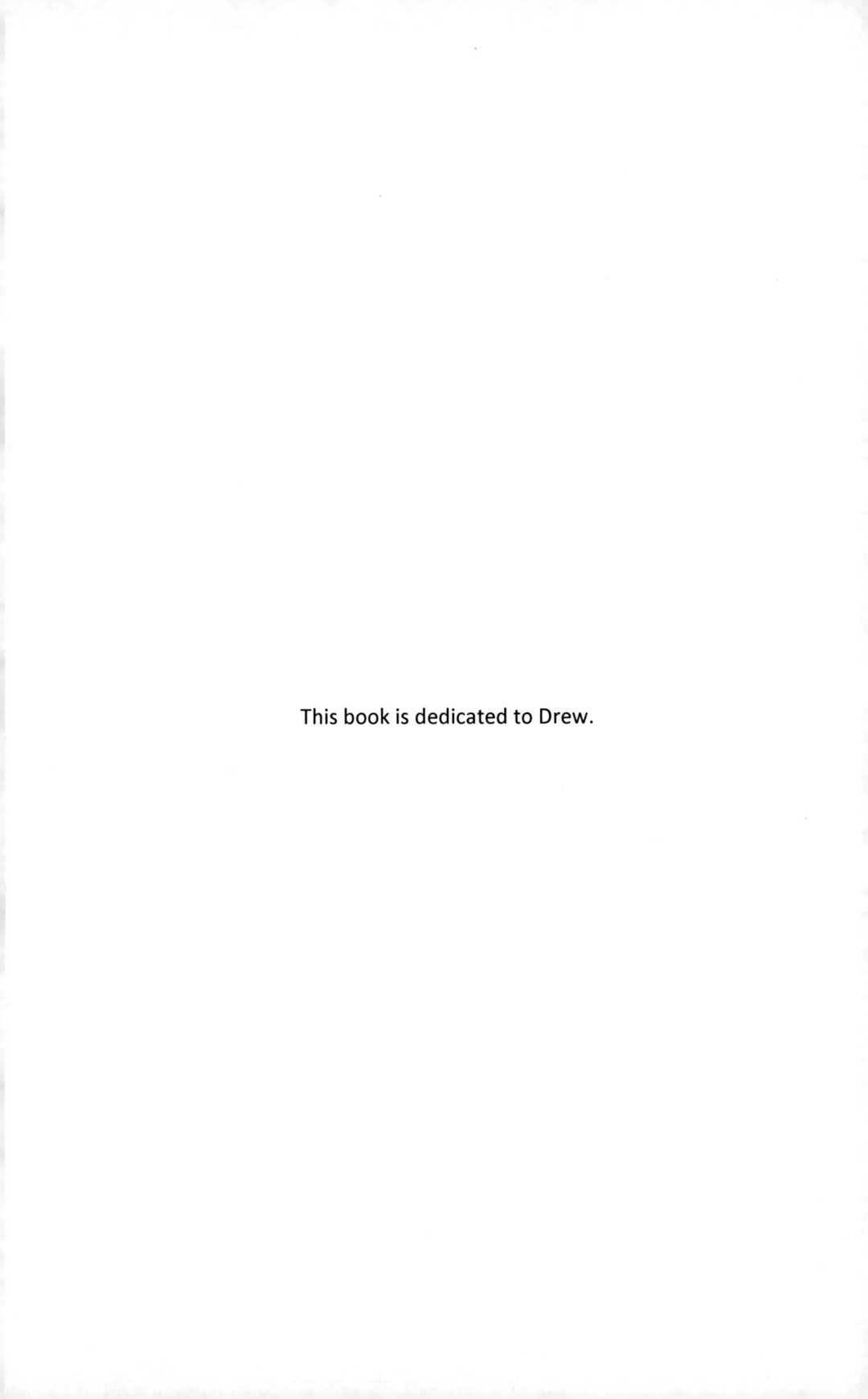

CONTENTS

ACKNOWLEDGMENTS

INTRODUCTION   1

ACQUIRING SOCIAL SKILLS

1. **Teaching Social Skills "Frontwards":** Teaching manners and appropriate behaviors before they're needed.   3

2. **Practicing Social Skills:** Repeated practice can achieve hard-to-get results in manners training.   5

3. **Teachers and Social Skills:** Social Skills can be as important as academics.   7

TAKING A POSITIVE APPROACH

4. **Listening to Yourself:** Listening to what you say to your children can help you communicate effectively.   9

5. **Sending Clear Signals:** Children with Asperger Syndrome need unambiguous communication.   11

6. **The Benefit of the Doubt:** The advantages of not leaping to conclusions.   15

7. **Taking Care Of You:** You can be a better care-giver if you attend to your own needs.   18

8. **The Power of Apology:** Admitting when we're wrong can gain our children's respect.   21

9. **Setting Smarter Goals:** Adapting your definition of success to accomplish what really matters.   23

10. **Rewarding Support:** Small acts of recognition can mean the world to people providing support to us and our children.   25

11. **Saying What We'd Want To Say:** Voicing the things we'd say to the people close to us if we thought we'd never see them again.   27

| 12 | **The Mojo Escape**: Relaxing and recharging your battery to deal with challenges. | 28 |

GENERATING AWARENESS OF ASPERGER SYNDROME

13	**Who's to Know? Disclosing Asperger Syndrome**: Determining who to tell about your child's diagnosis.	30
14	**Autism and the Pew Lady**: The danger of making hasty judgments about parents dealing with children's behavior problems.	33
15	**What's Wrong With Your Child?** Challenging destructive word connotations.	36
16	**Turning Students into Advocates**: Disclosing Asperger Syndrome to classmates to generate support.	39
17	**Liberate The Neurotypicals!** Educating others about Asperger Syndrome.	41
18	**Bullying and Tragedy**: Preventing bullying and its devastating effects on victims.	44
19	**They Know - Classmates and Asperger Syndrome**: Classmates can sense when someone is different. Knowing the reason encourages acceptance.	46
20	**The Benefits of Asperger Awareness**: How disclosure to classmates helped one boy with Asperger Syndrome.	48
21	**You Can Write A Grant Proposal**: Obtaining funds to increase awareness of autism and Asperger Syndrome.	50

FOSTERING SUCCESS AT SCHOOL

22	**Teaching Kids with Asperger Syndrome for the First Time**: Insights for teachers.	53
23	**Classroom Success Next Year**: Assessing your child's school year to make next year better.	57
24	**First Day of School Success Tips**: Steps parents can take to prepare for that big first school day each year.	60

25	**Innovation Likes Collaboration:** Generate better ideas and approaches by coordinating with others.	63
26	**Appreciating Teachers:** Great things teachers do to reach children who have AS.	66
27	**Empathy in the Classroom:** Encouraging understanding and acceptance in classmates.	68
28	**Today Is Going To Be Different**: A child looks forward to being accepted.	70

DEALING WITH ASPERGER SYNDROME

29	**Discovering Asperger Syndrome**: Using a diagnosis to face reality and improve family life.	72
30	**Asperger Syndrome: Difference or Disability?** Some odd behaviors are disabling – and some aren't.	75
31	**Different Means Different:** Understanding a child's different perspective and helping him succeed.	77
32	**Dealing With Kids' Setbacks:** Setbacks are part of the parenting process.	80
33	**Kids Need Each Other**: Including students who have Asperger Syndrome in the life of a school.	83
34	**Where's the Manual?** Discovering how to deal with your child's unique challenges and behaviors.	86
35	**Kids Count on Consistency:** Being consistent with children to get results.	91
36	**Learning Self-Advocacy Skills:** Teaching children to advocate for themselves.	94
37	**Get Real:** Doing an assessment of a child's strengths and challenges to help him progress.	97
38	**Meltdowns and the Big Picture:** Offers strategies for dealing with a child having a meltdown and those who witness it.	99
39	**Asperger Syndrome - Put Those Kids To Work!** Getting a part-time job can pave the way to a career.	102

40	**Writing Kids Off Is Not An Option:** Including children is important, even when it's inconvenient.	105
41	**One Size Fits One:** Finding ways to help students when standard approaches don't work.	107
42	**Knowing What We Don't Know**: How to avoid miscommunication in families.	110
43	**Rewriting Your Child's Script:** Redirecting children's negative thoughts.	112

SUCCEEDING AT PARENTING

44	**Becoming Bulletproof Parents:** Focusing on what's best for your child when he has a public meltdown.	114
45	**Cheerleading For Parents:** The importance of parents of children with Asperger Syndrome supporting each other.	116
46	**Reducing Special Needs Parent Stress:** The benefits of taking breaks to relieve stress.	119
47	**Listening To Your Kids:** Listening to your children can help ensure they listen to you.	122
48	**Teaching What Matters**: Teaching a child what he needs and can absorb.	124
49	**The Power Of Fun:** Creating a fun atmosphere can help families deal with difficulties.	127
50	**Being Who You Are**: Focusing on children's strengths to build confidence and self-esteem.	131
51	**Expectations and Best Days**: Having high expectations and a positive attitude can help your children succeed.	134
52	**Generating Good Surprises:** Consistently working with your child can prompt the behaviors you desire.	137
53	**You Don't Have To Go It Alone:** The benefits of support groups and counseling for parents.	139
54	**The Day Your Child Says Thanks**: Children who don't express appreciation today may surprise you with gratitude as they grow older.	141

| 55 | **Turning Failure into Success in the Fourth Dimension:** Reaching goals make take extra time for developmentally delayed children. | 143 |

IMPROVING FAMILY LIFE

56	**Stacking the Deck for Family Holidays:** Preparing to ensure your child with AS has a good family holiday experience.	145
57	**Grandparent Power!** Grandparents can provide wonderful supportive for children and grandchildren dealing with AS.	147
58	**Family:** Other people in the AS community can become "extended family."	151

TAPPING A MOTHER'S STRENGTH

59	**Asperger Syndrome and Mom's Secret Weapon:** Mothers need to give themselves credit for accomplishments they may not properly recognize.	153
60	**Feedback For Mothers:** Support for mothers who don't routinely get feedback from their children on the spectrum.	155
61	**Mothers and Belief:** Mothers who never give up on their children produce results.	157

BECOMING ROLE MODEL FATHERS

62	**Becoming Dad the Incomparable (A Father's Day Refection)** Carrying a picture of your child for inspiration.	159
63	**What's A Dad Worth?** The importance of fathers as role models.	161
64	**Dad Version 2.0:** Dads taking a more active role in their children's lives.	163
65	**A GPS for Fathers Day:** Dads learning about their children and father support groups.	165

HELPING SIBLINGS UNDERSTAND

66	**Autism, Asperger Syndrome and Siblings:** Children learning to understand and support siblings on the autism spectrum.	167
67	**Giving Siblings Their Due**: Making all the siblings in your family feel important as you're dealing with a special needs child.	170

LIVING AS ADULTS

68	**Adult Asperger Tactics for Parents:** An indirect approach may be more effective with adult children who have Asperger Syndrome.	172
69	**Future Prepping Your Child**: Determining your child's interests and aptitude to put him on a path toward successful employment.	174
70	**Preparing for a Car Accident:** A glove compartment checklist of things to do when you have a car accident for young adults with Asperger Syndrome.	177

Life in the Asperger Lane

ACKNOWLEDGMENTS

This book would not exist without my son, Drew. I've learned more about Asperger Syndrome from him than from any other source. My wife, Julie, has also played a major role in my education. Julie is constantly researching Asperger Syndrome and autism for our family and for the videos we produce. She routinely reviews my articles before distribution and makes helpful suggestions. She also often shares ideas for new articles. Our daughter, Jessie, has always been supportive of Drew, and of her mom and dad. So I'd like to thank my family for their support and for the positive examples they set that often wind up in my articles.

I want to acknowledge the many people who have generously shared their stories and their expertise about Asperger Syndrome with my wife and me. I'd also like thank the support group leaders and others who for years have distributed my writing. Having people tell me these articles have made a difference is one of my biggest rewards.

INTRODUCTION

Having a son with Asperger Syndrome changed my life. Being diagnosed with Asperger Syndrome changed it again.

My son Drew's diagnosis with Asperger Syndrome at age 14 helped my wife and me begin to understand this often frustrating, frequently funny, always interesting, and stunningly smart kid.

We threw ourselves into finding ways to help Drew. Julie's a designer. She designed solutions by researching Asperger Syndrome, tracking down conferences, joining and forming support groups and getting elected to the local school board.

I am, among other things, a writer and a video producer. Julie suggested we make a video to help Drew's teachers understand him. One video led to another. We learned from teachers, social workers, counselors, psychologists, authors, job coaches and others. We interviewed individuals with Asperger Syndrome and their families. We talked with bosses and coworkers of adults with Asperger Syndrome.

We discovered lots of techniques that we could try with Drew. Many were tremendously helpful. Time after time, Drew has exceeded the expectations we formed after his diagnosis and has blown past our fears. Would he ever make friends, learn to drive, have a girlfriend, graduate college, get a job, live independently?

Drew's done all that and more.

In 2003, I left my job in corporate public relations and we made creating videos about Asperger Syndrome and autism our full-time business. I started writing articles about what I was learning and distributing them to support groups across the country. The articles started appearing online and in newsletters and magazines.

I focus on the good stuff: practical things that I see making lives better. And the fun stuff. Everything goes better with fun.

I'm grateful to Drew for letting me share so much about his life. I'd routinely have him read an article that mentioned him before sending it out. I don't recall him ever censoring anything. He would correct me if I got the facts wrong about incidents that happened when I wasn't there. He even joked about being the poster boy for Asperger Syndrome.

I've collected the first few years of these articles in this book, and sorted them into categories. This means they're not presented in the order they were written, so you may read about Drew at one age in an article, and at a younger age in a later article. All these articles were written after Drew was diagnosed, but before I was diagnosed. I'll soon have enough articles for a second book, which will include writings about my diagnosis.

Because Aspergers can affect people very differently, I offer this book as a buffet. You can pull the points from each article you'd like try for yourself or your family.

By the time I was diagnosed in 2009, it wasn't a huge surprise. The diagnosis answered questions I'd had about myself my entire life, and explained why I'd often been able to relate to what my son was going through. Turns out I had the advantage of an inside perspective.

What I've learned in writing these articles has made life better for me and my family. I hope what you read here helps make life better for you and yours.

ACQUIRING SOCIAL SKILLS

1 TEACHING SOCIAL SKILLS "FRONTWARDS"

Why do we tend to teach social skills backwards? Instead of consistently teaching our kids manners, many of us wait until they do something wrong and then correct them.

Imagine using this approach in a driver's education class. They'd put you in a manual transmission car with no training. Then they'd turn on the engine and shove the car into the street, expecting you to learn to drive from the helpful suggestions yelled at you by other drivers.

Anybody think that's an optimal learning situation?

To give us parents the benefit of the doubt, we don't use poor teaching tools on purpose. We do what seems obvious at the time. But, looking back, I'm sort of amazed that I kept trying the same thing for so long when it wasn't getting results.

Even though I knew my son had Asperger Syndrome and that he had trouble learning social skills intuitively, for years I still tried to teach him by "correcting" him after the fact. Or rather, instead of teaching him, I corrected him. And got exasperated when he committed the same transgressions over and over again.

Well, I finally learned that if a door is locked, you have to try another one. In this case, the other door is explaining and demonstrating a social skill and having your kids practice it before they need it. And it pays off.

A little while back, I introduced my 20-year-old son to another adult. My son said, "How do you do?" He made eye contact and listened to what the person said -- and never once mentioned Star Wars. He even said, "It was nice to meet you," before he left. I thought back to ten years ago…when this conversation seemed like an impossible goal. But who was it impossible for? Once I tried the right door, the skill came through.

People with Asperger Syndrome can learn manners and social skills. Of course, how much they learn depends partly on their individual challenges and abilities. But it also depends on how we teach the lessons we want them to absorb.

I have a friend who tells a story about her son using a "script" he'd learned in social skills class when he happened to be seated next to a younger child on an airplane. As the mother of a child with AS, my friend was understandably nervous about how this would work out. It worked out great, because her son asked the other child a series of questions --and listened to the answers.

Hi, what's your name? What grade are you in? What's your favorite subject? Etc.

My friend knew this was a prepared script, but for the other child, it worked as a natural conversation. It helped the child with Asperger Syndrome interact in a comfortable way with another person – and it hopefully was a step toward helping the son learn more about conversation and preparing him to depart from the script.

Many of the manners and social skills we want our kids with Asperger Syndrome to learn can be taught, but we need to teach and practice these skills "frontwards," before they're needed. And practice is a key to success. A little regular practice time can help embed social skills so they become second nature to our kids.

There's no adequate way to describe how you feel when you see your son or daughter demonstrate good manners in the real world with no prompting from you.

Sometimes things are only temporarily impossible.

###

2 PRACTICING SOCIAL SKILLS

Does your child have Asperger Syndrome?

When's the last time you got frustrated because you told him not to do something, and two minutes later he's doing it again?

I think of this as "Teflon Shelf Syndrome." If you consider the brain as a storehouse with shelves, kids with AS seem to have some shelves that are coated with Teflon - and are tilted so things slide off easily.

So...it's not your son's fault that his finger strays to his nostril. It's not your daughter's fault she doesn't make eye contact when you speak to her.

But that doesn't mean you have to accept the status quo. There's a tool you can use to overcome problem behaviors: practice.

It makes good basketball players into stars. It gives musicians the ability to make a living doing something they love. It can give your child key social survival skills.

What is practice? It's training the brain and muscles to respond in certain ways. The brain is an amazing organ. People with brain damage have been known to retrain another area of the brain to take over the functions of the damaged area. If you think of someone with Asperger Syndrome as having a brain that's not damaged, but just wired a bit differently, there's a tremendous opportunity to "rewire" it with appropriate behaviors.

Of course, there's a catch. Practice takes discipline and patience. And because these are not qualities normally associated with Asperger Syndrome, you may have to supply them for your child. And we're not talking about discipline in the sense of punishment. We're talking about regularly making time in a busy day to do something that doesn't produce immediate results.

This "immediate results" thing is a real challenge. It's one reason many of us are overweight. We all know eating right and exercising could give us the buff bodies we see on TV. But it's just so easy to get distracted from that diet and that exercise when it takes weeks or months to see results.

Of course, it's different when you don't have any choice. Did you know Franklin Roosevelt had what he proudly referred to as "the arms of a wrestler" in spite of -- or rather because of -- his polio? Because his legs didn't work, he was forced to lift himself with his arms every time he got into or out of a chair, or a bathtub, or anything. Through all these small lifts, he developed tremendous upper body strength.

If you want your child to develop strength in social skills, you need to help him exercise those skills regularly until he masters them. Think of it as installing a rubber "gripper" strip on that Teflon brain shelf.

So, how do you start?

Start by writing down what's important to you. What are your overall social skills goals for your child? Now break those goals down into specific behaviors: Having David learn to use a handkerchief. Having Jennifer learn to wait her turn to speak and not to interrupt people in mid-sentence. Having Scott learn to answer a phone politely and take a message.

Set aside some time each day to work on a skill with your child. Keep your sense of humor and make the sessions as fun as possible. When one skill is mastered, start practicing another. Reward good performance with lots of praise.

If you can keep your sessions up for just one week, they'll become a part of your routine -- and much easier to continue.

Think of how your child may describe the sessions years from now, "My mom loved me so much she spent 10 minutes every day helping me learn to hold a conversation." "My dad worked long hours, but he made time every night to show me something about how to act in public. It sometimes took me lots of sessions to get one of his lessons, but he never got mad and he never gave up."

The biggest accomplishments don't always come from doing the big impressive thing. They can from doing the little important things -- everyday.

###

3 TEACHERS AND SOCIAL SKILLS

A while back, I wrote an article about having your first experience teaching a student with Asperger Syndrome. With so many teachers encountering students who have AS, I decided it's time for another chapter.

To illustrate both the positive aspects and challenges of Asperger Syndrome behaviors, I'll share an encounter that my son, Drew, had in high school. He was outside the school building waiting for his ride home, when he saw a guy he didn't know smoking a cigarette, standing with two other guys.

Drew impulsively said, "You know, smoking causes impotence."

One of the guys responded, "I don't give a F---!"

Drew, in full Asperger mode, shot back, "Of course not, you won't be able to."

This left the smoker speechless as his two companions collapsed in laughter.

While this sounds like a verbal triumph for Drew, it also demonstrated his inability to see that making a negative comment to a stranger was probably going to generate hostility. While he displayed his quick wit, what he said was not likely to make him any friends. It might even create an enemy, if the target for his humor felt the need to retaliate.

Still, it was a great line.

And it demonstrates how smart and funny a student with AS might be.

Or not.

Two students with AS can be as different from each other as any two other randomly selected students in your class. The thing they are most likely to have in common is difficulty understanding how to "read" others and interact as their peers do.

So one of the most important things a teacher can do for a student with AS is not academic, it's social. Helping these students develop their social skills is like giving someone with squeaking, sticking bicycle wheels a can of oil. Think of social skills as a human interaction lubricant that can help them succeed in the real world.

Academic success was never Drew's problem. His SAT scores would widen your eyes. But he was lonely early in high school because he couldn't seem to connect with classmates.

Then one of his teachers invited him to an after school Dungeons and Dragons game group where he met others with similar interests. Voila! He made friends. He's had a way to connect with others ever since. And success breeds success. The more a student with AS learns to interact with a few friends, the more capable and confident he's likely to be in dealing with other classmates. I think this teacher's influence played a role in Drew successfully asking a girl to his senior prom.

In college, Drew joined a D&D group and made new friends. After graduation, he took the initiative to form a group in our town that plays D&D and other games. The members of this group share other activities.

Drew is now working part time and has gone back to college to get a second degree. Developing his social skills has made him a lot more happy and confident. And it's a continuing process. Being able to interact was an important factor in getting his part-time job and it will be a crucial factor in getting a full time job in a tough economy when he leaves school.

If you're a teacher, you know that academics are important. But the things you do to help a student with Asperger Syndrome develop socially may be an even bigger life-success factor.

Oh, and avoiding cigarettes couldn't hurt either.

###

TAKING A POSITIVE APPROACH

4 LISTENING TO YOURSELF

Who do you listen to?

We generally listen to people we respect. Which makes it kind of ironic that we don't always listen to ourselves.

A few days ago, my wife pointed out an article about listening written last year by teacher Andy Dousis, who noticed his fourth grade students excluding a classmate from their activities. This classmate had trouble making conversation, so he sometimes pushed or grabbed others. He had other challenges, too, and often sobbed in frustration.

While the other students were initially patient with this child, they became less and less tolerant as the year progressed.

In looking at his own behavior, this teacher realized that the good example he'd set at the beginning of the school year had slipped away from him. In September, he had put considerable effort into integrating this "difficult" classmate into the class, and his students had responded. But as the year wore on and he'd gotten busier, he'd become impatient and spoken sharply to correct the child's inappropriate behaviors. The students were simply picking up their cues from their teacher. A good person and a good teacher, all it took to start fixing his approach was to listen to himself and realize what he was doing. Things got better for the lonely student and everyone in the class benefited.

This story brought to mind a conversation I had with a mother of a grown son with Asperger Syndrome at a conference in Philadelphia where my wife and I spoke. The mother explained how no one had known about Asperger Syndrome when her son was younger. She now looked back sadly at the way she had initially reacted to her son's difficult behaviors without meaning to. One day her four year old daughter, after continually hearing Mom speak sharply to her older brother, looked up at her mother and said, "If you'll be nice to Jim, I'll be nice to you."

In that moment, her world changed. Even before a diagnosis helped her better understand her son's condition, her daughter helped her listen to herself, and be more of the mother her son needed.

This mother wasn't alone. When my kids were little, my wife pointed out to me that I spoke to our son with AS in a very different, and less patient, tone than I used with our daughter. I confirmed this listening to myself on some home movies. It's easy to respond with the first thing that comes to mind to fix an immediate problem, but in a way you might regret later. I learned to change my responses.

This also was when I learned to patiently explain to my son how I expected him to act before he went into a situation, and even practice beforehand. The change wasn't instantaneous, but he did start doing much better. In fact, he'd often work hard to follow our instructions, then look up at us with an excited face and say, "I did it right, didn't I?"

This can be such a basic fix. Just listening to ourselves and making any changes necessary to say what we really want to say.

One of the best feelings in the world has got to be listening to yourself talk to a child, and liking what you hear.

###

5 SENDING CLEAR SIGNALS

My son is a careful driver. He uses his turn signals and appreciates other drivers who do the same – especially when he sees folks who don't. I appreciate products I have to assemble that come with clear instructions -- because I've wrestled with some that didn't. I also appreciate callers who leave clear answering machine messages — because I've had voicemail where callers rattled off a phone number so fast I couldn't understand it. I didn't feel kindly as I replayed the message again and again trying to catch the callback number.

I believe most of these communications transgressions aren't intentional. I think most happen when someone is in a hurry or distracted and absent-mindedly assumes that someone else knows what he thinks or intends.

Communicating poorly seems so obviously wrong and annoying when someone does it to us – and so innocent when we do it to others.

Like my son, I'm in the habit of using my turn signals, but there have been plenty of times when I could have communicated my thoughts more clearly.

It's easy to assume that you're communicating effectively when you're not. Say you're talking to a coworker about something your boss did, then you change the subject and start talking about a customer. After a while you get another sudden thought about your boss and say, "He really should have told us before he switched the schedule." Your coworker is confused because he thinks you're still talking about the customer. He didn't follow your mental process as it switched back to the earlier conversation.

Sometimes the problem is familiarity. I remember my wife complaining that she couldn't understand the instructions from workers at the department of motor vehicles where we used to live. After giving the same directions to people in line thousands of times, the workers rushed through them and ran their words together.

In one of my corporate jobs, our department bought a computer-controlled multi-media presentation system. The day we were scheduled to learn to use it, the trainer called in sick and they sent a sales person to fill in. As a teacher, he was a disaster. He ran through the instructions so fast that none of us could keep up. Then he got impatient because we weren't absorbing his information barrage. He knew the complex system inside and out, so its operation was obvious to him. He thought we just weren't listening hard enough.

As parents and teachers, we need to be careful not to make these mistakes with our kids and students. I've spent more than two decades in communications-related jobs, and I learned early that success isn't measured by what you do or say, but by what your audience absorbs.

With a new school year starting, parents can clearly communicate to kids that you have high expectations and that you're available to help them succeed. You can follow this up by helping your student get into the habit of having homework done before bedtime, setting out clothes, organizing backpacks and gym bags, and making other preparations. Of course, your focus should always be on helping your child take on these responsibilities himself. You also want to communicate to teachers that you take an active part in your child's education and that you need to hear promptly if there are any problems that your child needs to address — or any opportunities that might enhance his school year.

Teachers need to communicate their expectations to students and be clear about the kind of work and quality of work it will take to excel. It also helps to let students know how to ask for help if they're having trouble with the coursework — especially in ways that won't embarrass them in front of other students. Always posting assignments in the same place, handing out written instructions and posting assignments on a school website are good options to ensure students know what work to do and by what deadline. By providing clear expectations and instructions, you're serving as an excellent role model for them to follow when it's their turn to communicate.

When it comes to the nuts and bolts of communicating, here are some "best practice" tips I've picked up over the years that can help get a message across whether you're trying to connect with one person or a thousand.

THINK BEFORE YOU SPEAK. What does the person you're talking to know about what you're going to say? Is he familiar with it, or is the subject new to him? This will help you choose your words.

START WITH A HEADLINE. Headlines are designed to tell readers as much as possible about a story in the fewest possible words. Starting with a headline helps your listeners mentally prepare to absorb what you're going to say. For example, your headline might be: "Mom and Son Make List to

Shop for School Supplies." Next you translate your headline into real language and say to your son, "We need to go shopping for school supplies today. Let's make a list of what you'll need." This communicates your plans for the day much more clearly than musing aloud, "You can probably use last year's binders, but we need to get you some paper refills..."

USE INVERTED PYRAMID STYLE. This is a technique journalism students learn early. Basically, it means you put the most important information at the top of your story and the least important information at the bottom. That way, if someone only reads a part of the story — or if an editor cuts off part of your article, the readers still get the information they need most. When you're giving instructions, whoever you're talking to gets the same benefit if the first words out of your mouth cover the key points you want to make.

There are exceptions to this rule. For example, you may want to build suspense and then surprise your listeners for effect. But in most cases, your audience will appreciate your giving them the big picture and then filling in the details.

TREAT YOUR AUDIENCE AS CUSTOMERS. Thinking of your audience as customers can help you keep them interested by meeting their needs. Consider what they want -- and use it. Trying to convince teenagers to use good grooming? Appealing to their need to impress the opposite sex is usually a good tactic.

BREAK OUT OF YOUR RUT. If you routinely give the same instructions or information, it's hard to maintain your enthusiasm. Look for new words, or new methods, to deliver the goods. Finding fresh ways to communicate helps keep you energized and makes your audience more receptive.

BE CONCISE. It's easy to lose an audience. Saying what you have to say in as few words as possible can help you stay within listeners' attention spans and help them remember what you've said.

SEEK FEEDBACK. Watching faces while you talk or asking your audience for questions can help you make sure you're not wasting their time – or yours.

ENCOURAGE NOTE TAKING. If your message or instructions are long or complicated, taking notes can help your audience lock what they hear or see into their memories. People have better recall after they take notes, even if they never look back at what they've written.

To sum up, the next time you're about to communicate, put yourself in the position of the person or group that you're trying to reach and think,

- What do I really need to get across?
- How would I like to get this information?
- How can I be interesting, clear and concise?

As for turn signals, try thinking about how well drivers are communicating every time you see them using or neglecting their turn indicators.

Effective communications are always worth an extra thought.

###

6 THE BENEFIT OF THE DOUBT

People can be such jerks. Other people. Not you and me. When we get upset and are impatient or short with people, it's for good and valid reasons. If people could only see the pressures we're under or the unfairness of the situations we have to deal with... Hmmm.

I subscribe to a couple of special needs email bulletin boards. People share their experiences and I pick up some good ideas on how to understand and support my son who has Asperger Syndrome. Every once in a while, a few folks throw some pretty heated barbs back and forth. Someone takes exception to a comment, the tone of the responses escalates and then the accusations fly: "You're condescending!" "You're insulting!"

Yes, some of the "posters" on these boards bring some social interaction challenges with them. But I think it goes beyond that.

More and more, we find ourselves dealing with people we don't know – or don't know well. For most of human history, the vast majority of people didn't travel much and mostly had contact with the same group of people. I'm not suggesting there was ever a golden age of civility, but at least people had a better chance of understanding why someone was acting happy or sad or upset if they knew what was going on in that person's life.

We encounter so many people now in fragments of relationships. From strangers in an elevator to folks we "meet" on email bulletin boards to teachers in our kids' schools that we may see only a few times a year. Ever gotten mad about something and had that affect the way you dealt with people who had nothing to do with the reason you were mad? We all have. On the other side of the picture, it's easy to assume someone is reacting to us when he's actually got other things on his mind.

This all comes down to a simple observation. Things go a lot smoother when we give each other the benefit of the doubt.

In the bulletin board postings I mentioned, some writers read the worst interpretations and motives into what other people wrote. But others saw past the harsh words to the possible frustration and pain that could have sparked them. These pacifiers wrote to remind everyone that we're in these groups for mutual support and to give folks the benefit of the doubt.

These are people I admire. The ones who can look past their own experience to really try and understand what other folks are saying and why.

In the interest of full disclosure, I should mention that I'm not a natural born leader in this area. I've often found myself wondering how anyone could be so blind as to not see things the way I see them.

I look back on two experiences to help me remember to give folks the benefit of the doubt. When I was a young TV director new on a job, I met a co-worker who seemed to have an instant grudge against me. I couldn't understand it until a colleague told me about this guy's unhappy home life. I came to realize that he brought his problems to work and I'd walked into the line of fire. I also realized that I was the only one who could dial down the tension by not immediately taking offense when he was impatient and abrupt. We were never the best of buddies, but we did manage to produce some good work together.

While in that same job, I worked with an airline producing a video on "transactional analysis" to train flight attendants and reservations personnel to deal with upset passengers. The training divided interactions between people into three categories: adult, child and critical parent. When you interact as an adult, you're working from the facts and using logic. Conversations between two people acting as adults are pretty straightforward.

The training cited studies showing that when a person interacts in a childish manner (being selfish and whining) or as a critical parent (being condescending and scolding) – it's easy to be drawn into reacting in kind.

You may have seen emotional conversations like this, where one person is complaining and criticizing another and the other is either scolding back or is whining and making excuses. For example, a passenger might be so focused on letting the airline rep know how much a cancelled flight had messed up his vacation -- that he delays the rep from finding another flight that could salvage the situation. Then the rep gets upset and things go downhill from there.

The training encouraged airline personnel to always respond as an adult no matter what role a passenger took, because that's the best way to draw someone who's acting like a child -- or like a critical parent -- into responding as an adult.

It's easy to respond emotionally when we're dealing with issues affecting our kids or our rights or anything that really matters to us. But we're more likely to get a better outcome in the long run if we stay calm and deal with facts and not assumptions.

Maybe the teacher isn't ignoring my child's needs. Maybe she's got a plate-load of things demanding her attention and my child is just not her top priority. Maybe learning more about the situation and sympathizing with the teacher's challenges can help me find a compromise that's not everything I wanted, but workable.

Maybe the parent doesn't really expect me to ignore my other students and concentrate on his kid. Maybe I can use some of his ideas to help me teach his son and modify behaviors that might disrupt my class.

Maybe the person who made that outrageous generalization on a bulletin board isn't a dunderheaded jerk. Maybe he's someone who's had a painful experience that makes him over-react. Maybe in disagreeing, my response could start, "I look at that differently because…"

This is not to say that some people aren't dishonest or incompetent or prejudiced and that we shouldn't fight for what is right. Giving the benefit of the doubt doesn't mean giving in. It means withholding judgment until we have enough information to better understand where others are coming from.

We may find that storming the castle is absolutely the right thing to do. But if we do some reconnaissance before we sound the charge, we have a better chance of telling true opponents from potential allies.

As valuable as the benefit of the doubt is in dealing with relative strangers, it's a treasure to use with people we know well. My wife can testify that I'm not always world-class in communicating what I'm thinking and feeling and that sometimes I "over-assume" that someone knows what I meant to say. I'm guessing a lot of other folks are the same way. Think of bosses and subordinates, teachers and students, husbands and wives, parents and kids.

We all want to get the benefit of the doubt, so doesn't it make sense to routinely give the benefit of the doubt?

Especially, ahem, when you deal with me.

###

7 TAKING CARE OF YOU

A while back, I wrote an article urging parents of kids with special needs to deal with stress by taking breaks and finding other ways to relax. Given that I've been burning the candle at both ends with a blowtorch recently, I thought it would be a good time to revisit the subject.

While I usually follow my own advice, I occasionally...sort of...backslide and catch myself doing things that I know are counter productive. Hey, I'm human.

In this case, however, I've been able to keep up with taking breaks and relaxing with exercise since the beginning of the year, even through a series of stressful events. So, if you read the first anti-stress article and need a booster shot, this is my testimonial that taking some time for yourself pays off.

I did pretty good with breaks and exercise last year. But when my wife and I took on multiple projects in our business early in 2006 on top of the demands of family life, I risked getting sucked into the "non-stop work" vortex. This vortex was, too often, my daily life while I was in the corporate world. My wife has felt its pull for years, taking on the main role of dealing with schools and doctors for our two kids with special needs. I've talked with lots of special needs parents who know the vortex well.

Maybe getting a bit older has given me some perspective to help deal with its pull.

Whatever the reason, I'm convinced that continuing to make taking some personal time a priority in the face of demands and deadlines (not the top priority, but a priority) has kept me sane and in much better shape than I'd be in otherwise.

One of the best assets in my stress-beater portfolio is an early morning walk. For me, it has to be early morning. Once the phone starts ringing, getting away to walk is like trying to escape a black hole's gravity well. Walking early was a particular challenge because my wife and I tend to stay up late. There's always lots that needs doing and the next thing you know it's time for "The Daily Show" at 11 p.m. and we might as well stay up a bit later.

It's hard to stay up late and get up to exercise before the workday starts. One solution to this was taping "The Daily Show" to watch during lunch the next day.

I carry a small voice recorder on my walk to capture any good ideas or "to do list" items that my mind generates along the way. This way I can clear my head of them and deal with them later without stressing out that I'll forget.

Another benefit of walking daily and cutting down on my meal portions has been losing 20 pounds. You know those weight loss commercials that look so bogus? The ones where people go on a wonder diet, lose weight and tell you how much better they feel? Well, my wonder diet was just eating less, but the feeling better part is true.

I've seen a lot of people deal with stress. I've always admired the people who dealt with it well and tried to model their behavior. But it was hard to model someone who dealt with stress by taking time for himself when I felt guilty doing it myself. It's easier after you've given it a try and see that it makes you more productive.

Managing stress also can help you deal with other people.

When stressed, many folks tend to withdraw into themselves and focus on the task at hand. Without intending to, they risk being non-responsive or short with others. No surprise, this turns people off.

If you have a child with special needs, you can use all the support you can get. But if your reaction to stress is to withdraw, you may actually alienate people who could potentially help. This includes school personnel, friends, neighbors, relatives, and especially people you meet for the first time. Reducing stress can help you stay open to people and get help and understanding when you need it most. In addition to helping me keep fit, my walk helps my attitude.

I also take short breaks during the rest of the day. I figure that even if you have tremendous demands on your time, you deserve a bit of balance in your life. The scale may tip heavily towards your responsibilities, but if it tips too far, you risk falling over. And were would that leave the people who depend on you?

When you stretch yourself too thin, you also risk losing yourself and some of the best of what you have to offer the people you care most about. You can tell you've been lost when you suddenly find yourself again -- in a song on the radio or a line from a book or a movie. Maybe you're looking at a picture. But you hear or see something that shoots to the center of who you are and is instantly, recognizably special to you. At these moments, you touch some of the most valuable things you have to offer your family. Not just food and shelter and contact. Those parts that make you feel your worth as a person. Thoughts that generate caring and confidence and comfort.

It's easy to lose touch with them when you're stressed. A little relaxation can help you find them – and share them.

Your stress reducer may be different from mine. While I can recommend walking, I think almost anything you enjoy doing can be helpful if it gets your mind off your problems and lets you relax for a while and recharge your batteries.

Just remember, if it's your job to take care of everyone, that includes you.

###

8 THE POWER OF APOLOGY

When's the last time you apologized to one of your kids? Of course, maybe you don't ever do anything that requires an apology. If so, you are a very rare person.

I believe most of us can recall times when we've assumed something about our kids that turned out not to be the case. Other times, we may have understood perfectly well, but got frustrated and engaged in a bit of "scolding overkill."

I apologized to my adult son the other day after I jumped to a conclusion and assumed that he'd done something he hadn't.

I think there may be a tendency not to apologize to our kids (especially to younger children) as often as we should. Maybe we fear that admitting we did something wrong will undermine our authority. But kids can often sense when something's unfair. Do you respect someone more for not admitting a mistake, or for acknowledging it?

It's never pleasant to think about our sons and daughters discovering we're not perfect, but this is just not under our control. It's something kids figure out sooner or later. And how they think of us the rest of their lives depends, in part, on how they see us dealing with our imperfections.

Years ago, after I'd been working in public relations at a large corporation for quite a while, I asked an intern to proofread a news release I'd written. She gave it back to me without catching a typographical error I'd made. When I caught the mistake myself and pointed it out to her, she said she hadn't checked the document closely because I'd written it. She figured that with my level of skill and experience, her proofreading was just a formality. I had to gently disabuse her of the idea that people who have skills and experience don't make mistakes. In fact, the more experience you have, the more you learn to create safeguards to catch inevitable mistakes before they become major problems.

Given that I'm not perfect, I want my kids to see me as someone who's always trying to do the right thing. That includes owning up to blunders when I realize I've made them.

Sometimes, we can catch ourselves doing something we know is counter productive, but it's hard to stop. Like trying to change our kids' behaviors after an infraction by lecturing them at length and trying to make them feel really, really sorry.

How many of us have seen that loading on the guilt isn't effective in changing our kids' behaviors, but find it hard to hold back when we're caught up in the moment? I can claim to have gotten better at restraining myself, but it usually requires a conscious effort. Left to its own devices, my head often wants to administer a devastating dose of parental logic when a few calm words will suffice.

I'm a lot better than I used to be, but I still can go too far. When I do, or when I make some other family faux pas, I try and make it a point to apologize.

Unselfishly, this is a lot better for my kids in daily life. Selfishly, in the long run, this means they're more likely to think of me as a fair guy as they become adults. Not a perfect guy, but that was never really an option.

We won't discuss the number of times this means I have to apologize to my kids, my wife, and others. I'm not that good at math.

Sorry.

###

9 SETTING SMARTER GOALS

When you do a home project, does your child with Asperger Syndrome or autism get in the way? Let's say you're going to replace a faucet in your kitchen.

You ask your son to help. But he constantly complains about being bored.

When you ask him to go into the garage for a screwdriver, he forgets to come back and you have to go after him. When you ask him to hold a flashlight for you, he repeatedly gets distracted and lets the light wander. Your wrench slips and you skin your knuckles.

In this sort of situation, it's easy to get mad and lecture your son, or tell him he's not helping and send him away, or keep him by your side while you stew in silence, but vow to exclude him from your next project.

You don't go into the project intending to get impatient with your child or shut him out. Afterwards, you may regret the way you reacted. But you programmed your brain to accomplish a goal, to fix a faucet. Focused on that goal, your brain interprets your son's actions as interference, and you get frustrated.

What if you set a smarter goal? What if you define your goal as fixing the faucet while showing your son a good time? That programs your brain with a different set of expectations and you're likely to prepare and react differently.

Maybe instead of just pulling out your tools, you also assess your child's interests and capabilities before you start. You give him tasks that will interest him and prepare yourself to be patient if he doesn't do things perfectly. If he's younger, maybe you pull your tools from the tool box and have your son sort them. When he's a bit older, maybe you have him turn the wrench while you hold the light. If the job goes slower and isn't done perfectly, just adequately, your brain stills gives you credit for succeeding with your broader goal of making this a fun experience for your son.

Some parents do this intuitively. But the rest of us can do it, too. We just have to make a special effort until it becomes routine. It took me a while to build this into my thinking. But as I got better at it, my son and I started getting along better.

And, by finding ways to include our sons and daughters in small projects in positive ways, we help them learn practical skills and gain confidence.

Small things add up.

If you think of life as a race, we all get to the finish line one way or another. The real trick isn't winning at the end. It's finding ways to win every day, along the way.

###

10 REWARDING SUPPORT

Do you crave recognition?

Do you secretly yearn for praise of your accomplishments? While it's socially appropriate to be modest, just about all of us want our good works to be noticed. And we love rewards. What could feel better than someone praising us and offering a concrete expression of their appreciation?

During the years I worked in various corporate jobs, these expressions were frequently tangible. Company rewards often come in the form of plaques or promotions or bonuses. One of the best I ever received was a trip to Disney World with my family when my kids were little. Talk about making dad a hero.

Now that I'm working for myself, the rewards are different. It means a lot when customers praise the videos my wife and I make or when a program gets an enthusiastic review from an expert.

Living with less tangible rewards helps me appreciate all the other folks out there who provide support to children or adults who have Asperger Syndrome or autism and who don't have a formal reward structure. Folks like the moms and dads or siblings. Let's add grandparents, friends, teachers, tutors, counselors, aides, coaches, and therapists. You can't capture all the possibilities of people who should get credit in a list.

Some jobs, such as teacher or counselor, do sometimes offer structured, work-related rewards for providing excellent support. But in my experience, they usually don't reach the levels or frequency of the corporate cornucopia. And, trust me, many of the folks I've met who support people with Asperger Syndrome or autism deserve rewards just as much as my esteemed former corporate colleagues.

A while back, I wrote an article about the importance of giving positive feedback to the people we deal with on a daily basis. Now, I'm proposing that we take this a step further.

Think about someone who's made a difference in the life of your child on the spectrum and give him or her recognition AND a reward.

The reward doesn't have to be expensive. For example, as I write this, there's a framed document hanging on the wall next to me titled, "Five Reasons I Wouldn't Want Any Other Daddy." My daughter gave it to me when she was a lot younger. The five reasons she wrote are extravagant and funny and it's one of most treasured rewards I've ever received.

In an age of computers, it's relatively easy to create and print your own award citation. You can make up your own category and describe the great work someone's done. Pick up an inexpensive frame and, voila, you're giving a reward that announces your appreciation to everyone who sees it. But whether you offer an award plaque or cookies or a custom printed T-shirt, a tangible reward is a great way to give extra spark to recognition for someone who truly deserves it. Not to mention giving him or her that emotional boost we all need to do our best work.

Never underestimate the cookies. Rewards come in all sizes. And appreciation fills a part of us that should never go empty.

###

11 SAYING WHAT WE'D WANT TO SAY

My wife, Julie, and I lost a close friend recently. Bella died quickly and unexpectedly of a heart attack. It was a real shock. The kind that makes you look at your life and how you're living it.

Bella and her husband, Mike, were very close. So much so that it's hard to imagine one without the other. Mike told us that he only regretted not being able to say goodbye.

He didn't say he regretted spending too little time together. They shared interests and spent a lot of time with each other. He didn't say he wished he'd treated her differently. Whenever we saw them, they showed their appreciation for each other in all sorts of ways. Being with them was comfortable and fun. They were constantly building each other up. They were happy together and expressed it.

As much as Mike misses Bella, he can celebrate her memory without getting caught up in what he might have done differently.

Which brings me to the "looking at your life" part, particularly for those us with children on the autism spectrum who have behaviors that can be trying.

What if we closed our eyes and thought about learning that we might lose the people closest to us? Imagine the things we'd want to tell them. About how much we appreciate them. About the strengths they have. About what they mean to us.

Now what if we stopped imagining, and opened our eyes, and told them?

###

12 THE MOJO ESCAPE

Do you ever feel overwhelmed? Do you feel trapped by your responsibilities and yearn to escape?

Well, do it.

Not permanently. Just long enough to get your MOJO back.

Leading MOJO experts, who I just made up, contend that significant amounts of MOJO can be recovered by getting away from your worries for just a few minutes at a time.

The economic downturn has put even more pressure on parents who have their hands full supporting children with special needs. To someone already under stress, economic worries can seem to turn the straw that broke the camel's back into a bale of hay.

But with our families depending on us, we can't allow our backs to be figuratively broken. If you can't see a solution to a difficulty you've got, a short escape may help your brain approach the problem from a new angle.

Think of your brain as a muscle. You need to exercise it to keep it strong, but you also need to rest it.

I have a friend who started stretching his ankles so they wouldn't become painful on the long, daily walks he takes with his dog. But his ankles got worse. Turns out, he was wrapping a towel around the front of his foot and pulling it toward his knee for several minutes at a time. He found that the solution was to stretch for a count of ten, then relax for ten seconds, and continue that routine throughout the exercise. His ankles got better; because he gave his muscle fibers time to rest and recover between stretches.

You rest your brain at night, but it may need more time off when you're under stress. You just need to find the extra rest that will work for you. For some people, it helps to take short breaks during the day. For others, an evening out once a week doing something fun can be rejuvenating.

You may have to put some effort into making time for your breaks and covering your responsibilities. Perhaps you can watch a friend's children, and then have that friend care for yours. Maybe there's help available through a relative or a support group or church. It might help to make an appointment with your children's school counselor and ask him or her for ideas, or for contacts with other resources. If you're seriously stressed, you should consider seeing a doctor or other health professional.

Being stressed can block us from seeing solutions that others might help us see.

So, on your own or with help, consider finding some short escapes that can help you get your MOJO back. If that's too ambitious, just take off long enough to get your MO back, and leave a trail of breadcrumbs so your JO can find its way back when it's ready.

This is a time when your kids really need you -- and your MOJO.

###

Dan Coulter

GENERATING AWARENESS OF ASPERGER SYNDROME

13 WHO'S TO KNOW? DISCLOSING ASPERGER SYNDROME

Your son or daughter has Asperger Syndrome. Who do you tell? Who do they tell?

This can be a tough decision.

There are definitely two sides to disclosure issues. Personally, I'm in favor of being as open as possible with people who are going to have routine contact with your child – and that includes other kids. But it's an individual and family decision.

My son, who has AS, has gone through different phases. For much of his life, he's just wanted to fit in. And fitting in did not include telling other kids he had a condition with a weird-sounding name that affected his mental processes.

If your child's behaviors don't isolate him from other kids, this may not be a big issue. However, if the way your child acts drives a wedge between him and other kids, he has a dilemma. Does he keep silent about his AS and just deal with the teasing, harassment and isolation? Or does he tell the other kids and possibly make himself an even bigger target?

In this case, the problem is that the others already know something is different. They just don't know the reason. So not telling them the reason doesn't help your child accomplish his goal of fitting in or making friends or getting dates. But concerns about becoming a bigger target are real.

Kids can be unbelievably cruel. I recently interviewed a number of teenagers who have AS about their school experiences for a "peer awareness" video. It's amazing how some kids with AS can have such a positive attitude when you get a glimpse of the daily assaults on their self-esteem. Getting called a "retard" or being ignored can feel like a kick in the stomach. And some kids endure such treatment every school day.

You can't necessarily expect to change people who have their own problems and are intentionally cruel. But it's my experience that helping a group of kids understand a challenge or disability can improve your child's interactions with those who are not just plain mean-spirited. And if you can get the majority in the classroom to understand enough to avoid making thoughtless comments, and a few to actually reach out and be friendly with or to stick up for your child, you may dramatically improve his or her school experience.

The disclosure decision is up to you and your child. If you decide to disclose to a class, it helps to do some planning and preparation. It's important to involve the school and your child's teachers. Some parents choose to go to the class and make a presentation. Should your child be in the room when you tell other kids about AS? I think that sends a good message, but you need to see how your child feels about it. Some will want to be there and some won't.

Some kids even may choose to make the presentation themselves. Or, if standing in front of groups is not a strong point for you or your child, you may want to have a teacher, counselor or outside professional talk with the class. Just make sure that the presenter understands Asperger Syndrome and knows how it affects your child.

Most of all, I think it's important to give the whole picture and focus on the positive. You're not trying to get others to feel sorry for your child. You're trying to get them to see Asperger Syndrome as one of those differences we all have. If you choose to explain some of the "different" behaviors that the class is likely to see your child exhibit, be sure to focus also on his interests and strengths. The friendships my son has made have been largely based on interests he shared with others.

There's an interesting book by Norm Ledgin called "Asperger's and Self Esteem: Insight and Hope Through Famous Role Models." In this book, Ledgin identifies 12 historical figures and celebrities and cites evidence of traits they had that scientists now identify with Asperger Syndrome. Some of the people profiled include Orson Welles, Carl Sagan, Albert Einstein, Wolfgang Amadeus Mozart and folk musician John Hartford.

It's important to note that these connections with Asperger Syndrome are based on analysis and speculation and not everyone accepts this theory. Ledgin notes that "because these figures are all dead, we can never know whether all would have met the classic definition of Asperger Syndrome." It's also important not to set up expectations that everyone with AS should exhibit some form of genius. But, to me, the real power in the book is not that these people absolutely did or didn't have AS. It's that these people exhibited "different" behaviors and many succeeded in spite of some real challenges with social interactions.

I think you could consider a talk to a class about Asperger Syndrome particularly successful if you help a group of kids be more open to accepting others with a range of differences – not just AS.

My son is now in college and he's much more comfortable letting people know he has AS. Not that he feels it's necessary to tell everyone he meets. But he's learned that when he wants to tell someone, if he's open about it and doesn't act like it's anything to hide, people are more accepting. Confidence can be a powerful tool.

My son has spent a lot of time working on understanding and using the social skills that many people take for granted. But that's really only half the equation. We really need to educate people so that some quirky AS behaviors don't become a gate that locks others away from the positive things individuals with AS have to offer.

Who's to know?

It's a personal choice, but if you have Asperger Syndrome, letting the people you routinely deal with (teachers, classmates, supervisors, co-workers, etc.) know about AS and how it affects you can help them understand you, support you and appreciate you. And you may be making the way easier for the next person they meet who has AS.

The whole world doesn't need to know specifically who has AS and who doesn't. But who should we teach generally about Asperger Syndrome and other Autism Spectrum Disorders? Who should we show how to unlock the gate and accept some "different" behaviors to get the benefit of knowing the person inside?

Everyone.

###

14 AUTISM AND THE PEW LADY

I'm writing on behalf of the mother of a five-year old girl with autism and her mother -- and for me and my son. If you're not familiar with autism and you've ever wondered what you might do to help, here's a heads up.

I ran into the mother I mentioned at the Autism Society of North Carolina annual conference in Raleigh. She described how her autistic daughter had become upset in church and caused a small disturbance.

Let me note here that autism actually includes a range of conditions that fall under something called Autism Spectrum Disorder or ASD. People with ASD have a wide variety of challenges and abilities. Many forms of ASD are invisible, and you often can't tell by looking at a person that he or she has ASD.

Back to church. Some people with ASD can be upset by changes in routine. The little girl was upset because her Sunday school was cancelled for a special program in the sanctuary. She cried to the point her mother had to take her outside, leaving her two sisters behind. In the pew to the rear of the sisters, a woman's voice loudly proclaimed, "She's too old to be acting like a baby." This really upset the oldest sister and she had to be calmed down after the service by her mother, who told her that the woman didn't understand and not to let such people upset her.

Seeing the look in the mother's eyes as she told the story, I think the other woman was lucky she held her comment as long as she did.

What's one big thing can you do to help people with autism? Don't be the pew lady.

People with ASD often have problems with speech, or have trouble understanding explanations or difficulty expressing themselves. They may be hypersensitive to light or noise or touch or heat or cold. They may have obsessive interests and want to talk about them constantly. They may have unusual mannerisms such as hand-flapping or become upset at some slight change in their routine. They may lack tact and say things that are true, but socially inappropriate.

So, when you see a parent with a child who's acting volatile or eccentric, don't be too quick to chalk it up to poor parenting. You may be watching someone struggling to make the best of a very difficult situation. You'd never knowingly criticize a person in a wheelchair struggling to get up a ramp. Having a disability that isn't obvious doesn't make it any less real.

You don't want to be the pew lady. You want to be the person who understands the symptoms of ASD -- and that ASD is a neurological disorder that causes the brain to function differently -- and that people with ASD are not trying to be difficult -- they're often trying to overcome a difficulty.

And many succeed to amazing degrees. My son has Asperger Syndrome, an ASD condition that blew his mom and me away when he was first diagnosed because he was such an obviously smart little kid. Among other things, Asperger Syndrome gave him an obsessive interest in Star Wars and robbed him of the ability to instinctively understand what he needed to do to fit in with other kids. It also made it hard for teachers to shut him off in class. He'd learn the lesson, and more, and want to tell the class everything he knew on the subject. (Kids with AS are sometimes called, "little professors.")

Wherever we went -- the mall, our friend's houses, a museum -- our son was fascinated by objects and would obsessively pick up anything that caught his interest to examine it. He also had an intuitive understanding of mechanical systems, but that's another story.

We had questions: Would he ever "get better?" Could he control his obsessive interests? Would he ever be able to go to a mall alone, drive a car, have a girlfriend, live by himself, go to college, hold a job?

I'm happy to report, "yes" to all of the above. My son is now in college, living 3 hours away from his parents, a veteran of two part-time jobs and working toward a career in forensic science.

But whether people with ASD can go to college -- or it's a triumph to recognize their families' faces or dress themselves -- you want to be the person who helped make the triumphs possible. Even if that's by avoiding making assumptions or remarks when you see a child not "act his age" in public.

You want to teach your children not to tease or bully others, because teasing is torture to a child with ASD who doesn't have the ability to verbally fight back. You want to be willing to hire people with disabilities, because many make excellent, loyal employees at all skill levels. People with ASD often have strong skills in areas such as math, drawing, music or memorizing data -- and some have truly exceptional abilities.

You want to be the person who understands that one in 166 children born today has ASD and it's likely to affect the family of someone you know.

You're not the pew lady.

You're the person who's going to help make sure everyone with ASD is treated as you want to be treated: as a person who's not judged solely by a glance at his book's cover.

###

15 WHAT'S WRONG WITH YOUR CHILD?

My wife, Julie, and I were in church before the service recently and a woman came up and told Julie how nice it was that she'd brought our son Drew to their Sunday School class last week. "You really can't tell that there's anything..." She didn't finish the sentence, probably realizing how something like "anything wrong with him," would sound.

Her heart was in the right place, but her confusion demonstrates that we've got a ways to go in finding appropriate words and phrases to describe the challenges of people with Asperger Syndrome (which Drew has), with autism, and with similar conditions. I think, to her credit, she sensed that the word "wrong" wasn't appropriate.

And she was right. Yes, Drew has Asperger Syndrome -- and there's nothing wrong with him.

This is more that just simple semantics. It's complex semantics. The words we use to describe people color our perceptions. Many of the words used in association with neuro-biological challenges can be traced back to a time when people thought such challenges were a vengeful God's punishment for somebody's sin. If there's something wrong with you, it suggests you're different in a bad way – and you're separate from what's "right." The word "wrong" is also strongly associated with the word "mistake."

Our kids on the autism spectrum can be very different. Those differences can be difficult, even heart-wrenching, but the word "bad" doesn't apply. And our kids are not mistakes to be discarded, excluded or fixed. They're people with challenges. In that sense, they're just like the rest of us. Some just have higher obstacles to overcome and sometimes they have to find ways around these obstacles instead of climbing over them.

Too many folks see themselves as "us" and people with mental differences as "them." And they can pass those prejudices on to their kids. We've run into people who don't want special education kids associating with their kids in school because of fears the special ed kids might hold their offspring back. We've encountered parents who don't want school districts to spend money on special ed because they're afraid it might drain money from "regular" or "gifted" education resources.

Getting angry doesn't help. Or rather, what helps is to get angry enough to do something, calm down, and work to help people understand that we're all part of the same community. We'll all be better off when there are no "us and them" distinctions in our community and all the kids are part of "us." The fact is, we all benefit from projects and resources that help make people with mild or severe mental challenges become as independent and productive as possible. Just as we benefit from making typically developing and gifted kids as independent and productive as possible. These are artificial classifications anyway.

I've met lots of kids with AS who are also in honors or gifted programs. The bottom line is that it's in all our best interests to have as many of our kids as possible prepared to work and pay taxes and as few as possible on public assistance. Giving each child the assistance he or she needs now is an investment that will pay off for everyone, and it's right in line with the American philosophy of offering every child a free public school education.

The best way to foster that investment is to build a sense of community. To reach those folks who are receptive and to generate enough support to outvote folks who just don't get it and who can't see past their own immediate interests.

When I was a kid, I got a lesson in community that I couldn't fully understand until I was older. While in the sixth grade, my friends and I used to take "bike hikes" and ride out into the rural areas around Springfield, Missouri, where we lived. One day, a friend and I were biking through a neighborhood of a few houses on the outskirts of town. We saw a young man in his late teens or early twenties acting strangely. He was walking down the street, talking loudly to himself. Every few feet, he'd sit down and scoot a ways on his bottom. He looked dangerous to a couple of sixth graders.

My friend and I stopped at one of the nearby houses, told the woman who answered the door what we'd seen and asked her to call the police.

Her face full of concern, she looked down the street at the young man and told us that he wasn't dangerous, he wouldn't hurt anyone, and there was no need to call the police. He was her neighbor's son and she'd call his mother to let her know that he was outside alone.

I've thought of that woman from time to time and I increasingly appreciate the role she played in her community. She was an extension of the young man's family, caring about him and looking out for him. She was a good person. But more than that, she was a good person who knew her neighbors well enough to care about them.

I've run into a lot of caring people since that incident. Sure, I've also encountered people who are selfish and will never get it. But there are lots of people who don't understand enough to care because they just don't know enough about our kids. Chalk that up to a society where people move a lot, work long hours, drive places instead of walking so they often don't meet their neighbors, may have minimal contact with school teachers and staff, and may not even meet most of the parents of their kids' schoolmates. I think a huge number of these people have the potential to understand and care if we just give them a chance.

And while we're on the subject of understanding, reaching out to kids is particularly important.

As part of our business, we make videos that help students understand classmates who are different. Some of the most gratifying feedback we've received came after a psychologist used one of our videos in a school assembly to help educate students about Asperger Syndrome. After the assembly, a number of kids came up to a student who has AS and apologized for the way they'd treated him. For the first time, kids started sitting with him in the lunchroom and including him in playground games.

The assembly helped establish a sense of community at the school that was just as real as the community I rode into on my bike as a sixth grader. It was confirmation to me that we have to use every opportunity to reach for the best in people and help them see the big picture.

You can help by talking to other parents about what kids with "disabilities" are really like, by encouraging your school to make presentations on inclusion to students and teachers, by encouraging your PTA to make similar presentations to parents, by joining with other parents to form support groups and to lobby school boards to offer programs that help all kids -- including special needs kids, by actively supporting school bonds that include resources for all our kids, and by encouraging your local news outlets to do stories that show kids with challenges succeeding.

These are all important steps in the crucial job of helping people understand that kids can have all sorts of strengths and challenges and, at the same time, have absolutely nothing wrong with them.

###

16 TURNING STUDENTS INTO ADVOCATES

Do you get angry? I get angry. Oh, I'm pretty calm about most things. But when I hear about kids taking advantage of a child on the autism spectrum, my first thoughts involve swift and terrible punishment. Then I peel myself off the ceiling and think in more practical terms.

I felt a surge of anger today when I heard about a mother I know who picked her son up after school. He has autism and is in special classes, but eats with everyone else in the school cafeteria. As he got into the car, her son remarked that he was really hungry.

Why? Didn't he get to eat lunch?

No, he said.

It turns out the friend who usually ate with him had a schedule change, so he had to eat by himself. After he sat down, he realized he'd forgotten to get a drink. Leaving his tray on the table, he went to buy one. When he returned, someone had taken the tray. So, he went without lunch. Given the circumstances, it's a pretty safe bet his food didn't disappear out of good intentions.

As a dad of a son on the spectrum, it's easy to get angry and to want whoever took the tray to be punished. Of course, you'd have to find him or them. And have evidence they did it. And, you'd have to be careful that you didn't make the autistic student a bigger target in the future.

While I think it's appropriate to pursue individual tormentors after the fact, our broader goal should be to prevent such incidents. For example, suppose just one student had seen others taking the autistic student's tray and said, "Don't do that."

Looking back to when I was in high school, I was a member of a service club. We did things such as delivering food baskets to needy families at Thanksgiving and Christmas.

What a great service project it would be for any number of existing student organizations to educate their members about autism and Asperger Syndrome (and other special needs) and enlist them as advocates.

Most colleges look for community service in their applications. Being a special needs advocate is a service that students can provide as they go about their normal school activities.

Of course, having peers help peers is not a new idea. Quite a few organizations encourage students to support each other. One of the better known is called, "Best Buddies." Their website describes pairing children who have intellectual disabilities in one-to-one friendships with high school students.

If you can tap into a specialized organization such as this, more power to you. But enlisting the members of your school's existing student organizations and clubs could also have a tremendous impact.

Perhaps a psychologist, school counselor, or member of a local autism support group can make a brief presentation to each club. It will help if you can arrange for club members to be introduced to students who have autism or Asperger Syndrome (and who wish to participate) and learn about their strengths as well as their challenges. Then the club members' initial role might be as simple as to say, "Hi," when they pass these students in the hall, visit with them occasionally, and find ways to include them in activities. And, yes, to prevent bullying. These interactions could open the door to additional contacts and friendships.

Some schools make understanding and accepting differences an integral part of their programs. I'd love it if more schools took this approach. But I realize we sometimes need to start with smaller steps. Whatever you can do to help your school encourage students to be more understanding and compassionate is worth doing.

I know from personal experience about classmates who, after seeing presentations about Asperger Syndrome, apologized to students on the spectrum for how they'd treated them. A little education can also lead classmates to make a special effort to include and look out for a student they now see as a person, not just, "that weird kid."

The more students we can educate about special needs such as autism, the more we decrease the chances that one student will consider tormenting another. Or, if he does, the more we increase the chances that a third student will be ready to step up and say, "Stop."

Let's give as many students as possible the understanding to turn potentially demeaning and damaging incidents into actions that protect our kids and make us all proud.

That will be a lot more satisfying than getting angry.

###

17 LIBERATE THE NEUROTYPICALS!

Poor neurotypicals. Sometimes they just don't have a clue.

What's a neurotypical? It's a label for someone who doesn't have Asperger Syndrome or "AS." (I don't know who coined the term, but I first heard it used by Dr. Peter Gerhardt.) We can call neurotypicals "NT's" for short.

When an NT first encounters someone with Asperger Syndrome, he or she often sees quirky AS behaviors as a warning. "Opps, something wrong with this one. Better stay clear."

Many NT's routinely erect mental barriers between themselves and people with AS, without realizing they're walling themselves off from some really bright, interesting people. "Barrier behavior" can range -- especially in kids -- from avoiding or ignoring people with AS to taunting, harassing or taking advantage of them.

Let's call this Barrier Behavior Disorder (BBD). Unfortunately, BBD doesn't tend to fix itself. So who's going to break down these barriers and free the neurotypicals?

Um, that would be you and me. If you're reading this, you've probably either got AS, have someone in your family with AS and/or know a lot about AS. There's nobody more qualified to enlist in the NT-BBD liberation movement.

While I'm sympathetic to anyone with AS who doesn't want to widely disclose the fact, I also know of plenty of instances where neurotypical behavior changed for the better after someone took the trouble to help an NT understand Asperger Syndrome and what it does and doesn't mean.

It's natural to feel awkward when you're confronted with something new and don't know how to react. So let's tell neurotypicals a bit about Asperger Syndrome and explain how to react when a person talks obsessively about one subject -- or makes blunt observations -- or can't seem to ever find quite the right words to say. They'll be much more likely to interact long enough to see some of the strengths a person with AS has.

What I'm talking about goes beyond disclosure. I'm talking about an education campaign that can make life a lot better for all concerned.

You can start on a small scale. Are you concerned about what would happen if the police stopped your daughter who gets very upset with authority figures? My wife got a very positive reception when she held a seminar on Asperger Syndrome for local police.

Does your son shop at a local store? Maybe you could offer to do a quick talk on AS to a gathering of the store's cashiers just before or after store hours.

It helps if you keep your presentation short (you can do a lot in 5 or 10 minutes if you prepare properly) and if you describe specific behaviors and make suggestions about dealing with them. For example:

- If a customer is nervous and has a hard time finding the right words, it helps to be patient and friendly and don't rush the customer.
- If a customer doesn't seem to understand a part of the checkout procedure (for example, gives a checkout clerk his money before the item he is buying) just explain in a friendly way that you need to see the item he's buying so you'll know how much to charge him.
- Be careful not to talk to an adult or teenager having difficulties like you would talk to a small child, just explain things clearly in the same friendly tone of voice you'd use to give directions to an adult who didn't know where in the store to find the hardware department.

Of course, the idea for this education initiative didn't start with me. There are plenty of folks already out there helping neurotypicals learn about AS. But if you're new to the campaign, here's a tip: it helps to stress the benefits for both people with AS and for your intended audience when you're proposing presentations.

Most store managers, for example, should see the benefits of having their employees know how to deal with a situation calmly and avoid possible incidents where shopping is disrupted. Most police want to have good relations with the community and appreciate having accurate information when they deal with a person who has special needs. You're not telling people how to do their jobs; you're giving them information that will help them make good decisions in situations they're likely to encounter.

A father recently told me that his teenage son with Asperger Syndrome got upset anytime they were driving together and saw a police car. The father said he planned not only to talk with the local police about AS, but that he'd ask if an officer would be willing to do a practice traffic stop. After some preparation and discussion, the son could drive across a parking lot and an officer could "pull him over" and help him practice the right way to respond to a police officer in that situation.

What a good idea!

Which brings up another point. Asperger Syndrome support groups are great places to go for resources and ideas. (The ASPEN organization in New Jersey is an excellent example of an AS support and education organization. You can find out more information about ASPEN at www.aspennj.org.) If you're not the best public speaker in the world, maybe you can enlist another parent to help you make presentations. And maybe you can help the other parent in some other way.

There are also times when it helps to turn to a professional.

A mother recently wrote me about dramatic changes in classmate attitudes after a psychologist gave a presentation about Asperger Syndrome to a school assembly. The presentation helped the students understand what having AS was like and how kids with AS just wanted to be treated like everyone else. The mother said that kids who had routinely shunned and teased her son came up to him after the assembly to apologize. In the days the followed, classmates began including him in activities and sitting with him at lunch.

My wife and I have spent a lot of time with our son who has AS, helping him with his social skills and preparing him to interact with people in a variety of real-world situations. There are plenty of times where he's going to be out there and just have to cope. But anything he, and we, can do to help people understand what AS means and meet him halfway tends to level the playing field -- so he's not fighting barriers that shouldn't be there in the first place.

It's sometimes amazing how great people can be if you just let them know what's going on and give them a chance.

So let's all work to eradicate NT-BBD.

Our neurotypical friends deserve nothing less.

###

Dan Coulter

18 BULLYING AND TRAGEDY

This week, thirty-two people died at the hands of a disturbed student at Virginia Tech. Thirty-three people, when you also count his suicide.

I was struck by statements from a number of people who had responsibility for comforting the friends and family of the victims. They said there was no one particular thing you could say. Often you just needed to be there to listen. I think that's wise counsel. This is a searing, unimaginable loss, felt in his or her own way by every person in mourning. My heart goes out to them.

What I know of this tragedy comes from media coverage. As usual after such an event, much of the coverage I've seen tended toward the sensational, but portions may help us understand some useful things about what happened.

I saw an Associated Press story today by Matt Apuzzo. It quoted former classmates of the killer, Cho Seung-Hui, describing how Cho was bullied and teased in middle school and high school.

In the story, a classmate described an incident in high school when Cho remained silent, looking down after an English teacher had called on him to read aloud in class. When the teacher threatened him with an "F" for participation, Cho began to read, but used a strange, deep voice.

"As soon as he started reading, the whole class started laughing and pointing and saying, 'Go back to China'," recalled a student who'd gone to high school with Cho.

Another former classmate described students in middle school who were "really mean" to Cho, pushing him down and making fun of the fact that he didn't speak English well.

While this is only part of the picture, it seems clear from the writing and videos Cho left behind that being bullied and harassed had a terrible impact on him.

I wonder what people will take away from this.

I hope they don't start seeing everyone who is bullied as a potential mass murderer. Something else that comes out of the coverage is that Cho was treated for mental illness and had lost touch with reality.

But I hope people do see the anguish that bullying and teasing can cause.

I've heard again and again from parents about children robbed of any joy at school. Kids who just want to be accepted and "treated like everyone else."

Who suffer stomach aches from the fear of being preyed on. Kids with tremendous potential being made to feel like nothing.

And yes, there are some kids who bullying may push toward violence.

If you've watched the news coverage about the Virginia Tech tragedy, you've probably heard commentators and experts talking about what we might do to prevent such attacks in the future. I've heard suggestions about profiling, increased campus security and a range of other options.

But one practical thing we can all do, is work for anti-bullying programs that educate both students and teachers in our schools. While such programs can help millions of students who wouldn't harm anyone, one also might touch a life in a way that could help avert a tragedy in the making.

In addition to mourning the lives lost at Virginia Tech, working to enrich and preserve lives in the future is a memorial available to us all.

###

Dan Coulter

19 THEY KNOW: CLASSMATES AND ASPERGER SYNDROME

I've heard it too often. The teasing and rejection that many children with Asperger Syndrome face in school from classmates who don't understand why they act different. The frustration and impatience from teachers who assume that these students are simply being disrespectful, stubborn, or lazy.

I've also often heard about how much things have improved for children with Asperger Syndrome when teachers and classmates learn about AS.

Parents who were concerned that they'd make things worse for their children if they disclosed the facts, have told me how those disclosures made things better.

If you're the parent of a child with AS worried about what will happen if other students find out, here's a thought: they already know.

They know they have a classmate who has different and difficult behaviors. But they don't realize the reasons. And the reasons they imagine are much worse than the facts.

So children who have AS are routinely misunderstood by unprepared teachers and classmates. Their school lives can be torture. They're friendless and under constant stress. No matter how hard they try, they can't make things better. Often, they don't tell parents the worst of it. From shame, or because they stop believing anything can be done for them.

Disclosure may not be the best approach in every situation, but I'd urge parents to consider it carefully before ruling it out. Again, I've heard stories of dramatic improvement from parents who've chosen to share information about their children's condition with school staff and classmates. Children making real progress with help from patient teachers. Children making friends for the first time and being invited to parties. Children being protected from bullying by other students. Children leading class sessions on topics of special interest or tutoring other students. Children feeling like they belong.

I recently heard from a father who said, in addition to the many other benefits of disclosure, that the parents at his son's new school don't treat him and his wife like they're the worst parents in the world.

I'd love to have us all make 2009 the year of Asperger Syndrome awareness.

You can get help making decisions about disclosing AS from support groups, school counselors, or psychologists who specialize in AS. The magic is not simply in telling others your child has Asperger Syndrome. The magic is in sharing appropriate information in a way that allows them to understand your child's thought processes and shows how they can make allowances and help him interact and progress. It's also important to talk about your child's strengths and what he has to offer, and not focus only on his challenges.

A mother just wrote me to ask how old classmates need to be to understand about Asperger Syndrome. Great question. In the youngest grades, you may determine that you don't need to discuss the diagnosis. Maybe you just address behaviors. Everybody's brain works differently. Jared is very enthusiastic. He has trouble remembering to take his turn and raise his hand so we need to be patient with him. Emily is smart, but she has trouble remembering to be polite. She doesn't mean to hurt your feelings when she says things about how you look. We need to tell her when she says something that hurts our feelings so she can learn how friends talk to each other.

You need to make determinations about what to say based on your child and his or her classmates, but I think the earlier children hear the words Asperger Syndrome and what AS does and doesn't mean, the more accepting they're likely to be from that point forward. And children are never too young to learn that we're all different and that we need to treat each other with patience, kindness and understanding.

If you're the parent of a child who has Asperger Syndrome and you're conflicted about disclosing his or her condition to teachers and classmates, consider how great it would be to feel relieved and glad that…they know.

###

Dan Coulter

20 THE BENEFITS OF ASPERGER AWARENESS

I've written quite a bit about the benefits of disclosing Asperger Syndrome. My wife and I got an email last week that really drove the point home.

The email came from a mother who, years ago, worked with her son's psychologist to schedule a middle school assembly about Asperger Syndrome. The psychologist used one of the DVDs we produced to help the school's students understand something about AS behaviors and what caused them. After the assembly, this mom wrote us to tell us how students who'd formerly ignored or teased her son had become his supporters.

In her recent email, she said her son is now in high school and has several friends. He's starting the college search process and she asked about college programs for students with Asperger Syndrome. She said her son sometimes runs into boys he knew in seventh grade and that they continue to be interested in him and how he's doing. She mentioned that these former classmates still have memories of the video and the experience.

Of course, this email made us feel great. But our video was only one part of this success story, which was created by a student and parents willing to disclose, an enlightened school staff willing to hold an assembly, and an effective communicator willing to interact with the students.

We've also heard success stories about the children who've been in our videos. A number of parents have asked about opportunities to have their children participate in new videos to show how much progress they've made. We know some of these parents well enough to see what a huge role they've played in that progress. These parents are solid advocates for their children and are raising them to be as strong, confident and independent as possible. Being open about Asperger Syndrome sends a strong message to these children about their self worth, just as they are.

Disclosing that a child has Asperger Syndrome should always be a personal and family decision based on your circumstances. But it's one I urge every parent of a child of with AS to seriously consider.

We're now working on a DVD to help people with Asperger Syndrome find and keep a job. We're interviewing successful job holders with AS, as well as their employers and job coaches. In an environment where unemployment is dramatically high for people with AS, all of these employees have been working steadily for years. Every successful job holder we've interviewed has talked about the importance of disclosing AS to supervisors and co-workers. This helps people see past their AS behaviors to appreciate their strengths and productivity.

It's something to think about. Children with Asperger Syndrome grow up and need to find work just like everyone else. Continuing disclosure may be an important factor in your child's lifelong success.

Lifelong success. That has a nice ring to it.

If disclosure is a building block to lifelong success, shouldn't we start laying the foundation as soon as possible?

###

Dan Coulter

21 YOU CAN WRITE A GRANT PROPOSAL

Get a grant. It's free money.

Okay. Not totally free. You do have to so some work for it by researching and applying. And you'll be almost surely be competing with others applying for the same grant. That being said, if you have good idea for a project to help others, there are literally millions of dollars out there waiting to be allocated to deserving projects.

Write a strong proposal, and you could receive all the "free" money you need to accomplish your goal.

I recently took a course in grant-writing taught by someone who's written a lot of successful grant proposals. I'll share some of what I learned.

Let's say you want to take on a project that's close to my heart, getting a grant to help educate students about classmates who have Asperger Syndrome or a similar autism spectrum condition. Good for you. Here's how to proceed:

First, set a specific goal. For example, do you want to educate all the students in a school or in a school district?

1. Determine ways to accomplish your goal. Maybe you want to provide an hour of instruction to every student in your target audience.
2. Seek out individual grants that are a good fit for your project. Grants are offered by governments, private companies, foundations and other groups. You can search for U.S. government grants on www.grants.gov. Remember, that's ".gov" and not ".com." Another good source is www.foundationcenter.org. Consider also applying to local companies which have a stake in your community. Even companies that don't routinely offer grants might be interested in funding your project. Here's a great tip: some of the best sources of accurate, up to date information about available grants are routinely published in lists. While these lists can be very expensive, you can access them for free in many public libraries. Call your local library and ask if they have a Non-Profit Resource Center. If so, stop by

and do your research there. A helpful reference librarian can speed your search. CAUTION: if you do an Internet search for grants, you're likely to find lots of organizations interested in charging you money to provide lists of grants that you can apply for or to write your grant for you. Some of these offers are likely to be rip-offs. I'd avoid them and do your own research and writing.

3. When you find some promising grants, read carefully over their requirements. Some grants are available to individuals. Some are limited to schools or non-profit organizations. A grant's written requirements should help you determine whether you qualify to apply. Many funding organizations offer websites where you can find details about their grant requirements, see what they've funded in the past, and sometimes even fill out a grant application online.

4. After you've done your research, write your grant proposal. Follow the guidelines of the funding organization carefully. These will vary, but many organizations use these categories:
    a. Executive Summary: An overview of your request.
    b. Statement of Need: What needs changing and how you intend to change it.
    c. Mission Statement: What your organization strives to do.
    d. Vision Statement: What the world will look like when you accomplish your mission.
    e. Management Team and Competencies: A description of the people who will work on your project and their qualifications.
    f. Project Description: What you are going to do to meet the need you described in your "statement of need." This is the heart of your proposal.
    g. Project Evaluation: How you will measure your results.
    h. Organization Budget/Financial Statements: Financial information about your organization, if you are applying on an organization's behalf.
    i. Project Budget: What funding you need and how you're going to spend it.
    j. Other Attachments: Different organizations may ask for additional information.

As you're writing your proposal, remember it has to stand on its own. You won't be there to explain it when it's read. Share your finished proposal with some friends or colleagues and get their feedback. If they don't understand parts of your proposal, rewrite those sections so they are more clear.

This is a general overview of grant proposal writing. For an Asperger Syndrome/autism awareness project, you might ask for funds to have an expert prepare materials to use in age-appropriate presentations that will be used with children throughout a school system. Your expert might train teachers to make in-class presentations or to lead class discussions after the expert makes a presentation in a school assembly. These presentations would be designed to help classmates understand and support children that they previously teased or excluded from activities because of their behaviors.

It's important to include funding for measurement. You might survey student attitudes toward classmates who think and act differently and what they know about Autism Spectrum Disorders before, and then again after, your presentations. Remember, capturing evidence of success can help you when you apply for your next grant.

And you don't necessarily have to start from scratch with your presentations. You may choose to use grant funds to purchase an existing program and associated materials.

For example, The Anne Arundel County Public School System in Maryland, USA has developed an Autism and Asperger Syndrome awareness guide for elementary schools. The guide is called, "Building Bridges - A Multidisciplinary Team Approach to Supporting Students with Asperger's Syndrome and Autism in the Classroom." The school system has information about the package available on its website: www.aacps.org

Whether you prepare your own materials, or buy an existing package, a grant could help a school or a school system dramatically improve the lives of their students with autism spectrum conditions. And, at the same time, teach their classmates valuable lessons about accommodating differences in an increasingly diverse, global workplace.

There may be no free lunch. But there is free money available. And if you have to work for it through research and grant proposal writing, it still could be the best bargain a student body could ever hope for.

###

FOSTERING SUCCESS AT SCHOOL

22 TEACHING KIDS WITH ASPERGER SYNDROME FOR THE FIRST TIME

You're a teacher. You've just found out that you're going to have a student with Asperger Syndrome (AS) in class this year. You're in for an interesting year. And that's not coded language for "brace yourself." It's a real-life perspective that teaching a child with AS often gives you as many opportunities as challenges.

First, the nuts and bolts stuff. Asperger Syndrome is a neurobiological disorder on the higher functioning end of the autism spectrum. It's an increasingly common diagnosis and many kids with AS are in regular school classes.

Kids with Asperger Syndrome can have a variety of symptoms and behaviors, but they generally have problems with social and communications skills. That's only half the story, though. They also typically have IQs in the normal to very superior range. Asperger Syndrome has sometimes been described as "little professor" syndrome, because often kids with AS become walking encyclopedias about topics that interest them. And therein lies one of the biggest problems for these kids. Many look so normal and are so advanced in some ways that it's hard for people to understand why one can't read a teacher's facial expression, or another has trouble making eye contact, or a third takes expressions literally and misses implied meanings.

It can be tough to fathom why a child who has an extensive vocabulary and knows the material you assign inside out can't seem to hold a casual conversation with a classmate.

Here's the good news. You can often build on that child's strengths to help him modify his "out of the norm" behaviors and make a lot of positive contributions to your class.

That's really the bottom line for you: finding ways to make the year a good experience for every child in the room, including the one with AS -- and, of course, for you.

You can't discount your needs in the process. So let's make them a priority, too. First, you may want to learn a bit more about Asperger Syndrome. One of the most user-friendly sources is the www.aspennj.org website. It's run by a non-profit "education network" with a lot of clear, easy to access information. Their "What Is Asperger Syndrome?" page is a great concise overview of AS. Your school counselors may also have information or may be able to put you in touch with other teachers who've had experience with AS.

Once you understand a bit about AS, a child's parents often can help you understand how it affects him or her. You're not asking them to tell you how to teach, you're looking for accurate information that can help you determine ways to successfully direct and motivate their child. You and the parents may even be able to cooperate to identify behaviors a child needs to work on and reinforce them at home and at school.

For example, many kids with AS are impulsive. You may teach a student who loves class participation, but has trouble sensing when she should stop talking and give someone else a chance. You might work out some signals that only the two of you and her parents know (like putting your hand to your chin as if you're considering what's being said or walking to stand right in front of that student's desk) that cue her it's time to stop talking. If you have a student with AS who is especially eager to participate, you may want to routinely call on that student first or second, so he isn't coming out of his chair in his eagerness to contribute.

Kids with AS often need structure and respond best when they have clear, consistent direction. Some teachers find it works to write the homework on the blackboard in the same place every day, announce tests well in advance and routinely remind the class of the dates when longer term projects are due. Such techniques usually benefit the entire class.

There are lots of specific things you can do, but the most important thing is your approach. Your approach is the magic bullet that can help the entire class learn one of the lessons that matters most to all of us: how to accept and get along with a variety of people.

When I was in elementary school, we had a category on our report cards called, "citizenship." There are all sorts of outside pressures that tear at the kind of behavior that got you an "A" is citizenship. TV commercials routinely encourage viewers to be greedy with their products. The message: if you want to be cool, keep the best stuff for yourself -- people who care about other people are suckers. Commercials that target kids also talk a lot about having "attitude," in a way that confuses confidence with arrogance and selfishness. Comedians casually toss around the word "retarded" as an insult.

Teachers can serve as a powerful role model to counteract these negative influences. Having a child with Asperger Syndrome in your class gives you the chance to show your students that people who have challenges can also have strengths. That in looking past someone's quirks, you can find someone worth knowing. That life is richer if you don't solely interact with kids who are like clones of yourself.

Academics can be a bridge. My son has Asperger Syndrome and was not sought after for teams on the playground. But back in class, kids would eagerly seek to get Drew on their academic teams because he routinely knew the right answers. That's not to say every kid with AS is an academic whiz, but most have special interests and strengths.

The first signal to a class on how to treat a kid with Asperger Syndrome often comes from the teacher. If students sense that a teacher is impatient and critical of an AS student's behaviors, it's like declaring open season to ignore or tease him -- in and out of class. Approach that student with patience and respect, and you've set that tone for everyone else. It can mean the world to some kids with AS just to have other kids say, "Hello."

One of the key issues you may face is helping a student tell the rest of the class about Asperger Syndrome. Whether or not to disclose a disability is a decision for the student and his parents. If they decide to tell the class, you can play an important role in treating AS as just another one of those differences that we all have. In my experience, other kids are more likely to give a student who has some odd behaviors the benefit of the doubt if they know the reason.

A student might choose to talk with the class himself about AS, or his parents might make a presentation or bring in a psychologist or other expert. Some kids with AS want to be in the room for such a presentation and some don't.

If you take part, here's a tip I picked up. It's a good idea to write "Asperger Syndrome" on the board and pronounce it for the class right off the bat. This makes it less likely that some comic in your class will hear the name as "Ass Burger" and have a field day with it. You might even mention that the condition is named after a Viennese doctor named Hans Asperger who identified the syndrome more than 50 years ago.

I find kids are interested to know that Dan Aykroyd from Saturday Night Live said in an interview on National Public Radio that he has Asperger Syndrome.

There's a fair amount of speculation that people such as Thomas Jefferson, Albert Einstein, Wolfgang Amadeus Mozart, and Isaac Newton had AS. Even though no one can prove historical figures had the syndrome, I think it's fair to note that these folks all had documented behaviors which are common to people with AS. The point is not to suggest that every kid with AS is a genius, but that people with AS can have a range of talents.

Having a kid with Asperger Syndrome in your class may be the greatest opportunity in your career to change a student's life for the better. My son's about to head off for his senior year of college, and my wife and I always enjoy getting the chance to visit with some of the great teachers he's had along the way to let them know how he's doing – and thank them.

Here's thanking you for reading this article and for being interested in helping that kid in your class who needs something extra to make it.

He'll remember you.

###

23 CLASSROOM SUCCESS NEXT YEAR

Do you want next year to be different?

If you want the coming school year to be better for your child with Asperger Syndrome, whip out a sheet of paper. Now, let's do a review of what worked this year and what you'd like to see carried over into next year.

What did Jimmy like about school? What did Mary do best in? What did the teachers do that worked? What did you and your child do that worked? What do you want to make sure you capture and repeat next year?

Okay, now for the dark side. What didn't work? What do you really want or need to change? The first step is to write out what the problems were, then brainstorm about what you can realistically do to make next year different – and better.

Keep in mind actions that you and your child can take over the summer, such as social skills training.

Probably the single most important external factor affecting how your child does in school is his or her teacher.

The best teacher-student matches for kids with Asperger Syndrome tend to be instructors who have a lot of structure in their classroom, but who are also flexible. Structured but flexible? This is not a contradiction.

Here's an example. Mr. Johnson's a math teacher who always has the day's homework assignment written on the board. He gives clear instructions and due dates when he assigns projects. He has a quiz every Wednesday and a test every Friday.

While Mr. Johnson provides structure, he understands that Jack (who has AS) has a problem wanting to talk at great length whenever he answers a question. Mr. Johnson is willing to work with Jack on signals just the two of them know that help Jack realize it's time to stop talking and give someone else a turn. In other words, Mr. Johnson provides the structure that Jack needs to understand the assignments, but he's also flexible enough to accommodate and help modify some of Jack's Asperger Syndrome-related behaviors to help him learn and minimize class disruptions.

So, how do you get your child into a "Mr. Johnson" class?

Strategy.

First, talk with your school counselor, principal or other appropriate school official about student-teacher assignments. Schools do this at different times: before this year ends – during the summer – at the beginning of the next school year. Whenever your school makes these assignments, it's best to get your input in early.

Take your list of what will help your child learn – and what will hinder learning – when you talk with your school contact. Your approach is that you want to provide the school input for their teacher selection. Things tend to work best if you don't ask for a specific teacher or teachers. Show the school that your child will learn best – and have fewer problems that could result in class disruption – if he is matched with teachers with certain attributes. Then list the attributes and the advantages.

You're a salesperson, showing the school contact why it's in the school's best interest, as well as yours, to make a good teacher-student match. If the school has already made a match that doesn't look workable, this approach could help convince them to change things around before the school year starts. It's in everyone's interest to have the year go smoothly.

Once a teacher is selected, move heaven and earth, Mars and Pluto to get a meeting with the teacher (or key teachers if your child has more than one) before the school year starts. At that meeting, offer information to help them understand your child and make things go smoothly. You're not telling them how to do their jobs, you're providing information they can use to make decisions.

Always counsel from consequences -- and experience.

"Andy really responded well when his teacher called on him first or second." "Sally tended to get very upset when her teacher had the students pick their own cooperative learning partners." "Kumar has tended to learn best when his teachers have used visual aids and the lessons weren't purely verbal."

Be careful not to overwhelm teachers with information and don't forget that your child is only one of a classroom full of kids that a teacher will need to manage. Teachers tend to be stretched very thin these days. Some students with AS have the help of in-class special education teachers and aides, but many are in classes with one teacher at the front of the room. Ask the teacher to call you if problems arise and not to wait for regularly scheduled parent-teacher meetings.

You may need to educate a teacher about Asperger Syndrome, but don't offer a stack of books. Start with a single article or video that a teacher can read or view in less than an hour. (My wife and I made a 44-minute video for this purpose after having to explain our son's AS to new teachers each year.)

Most teachers tend to appreciate your sharing information with them if you take the right approach. It's a mixed blessing that there's a dramatic increase in cases of Asperger Syndrome being diagnosed. No one wants more kids to have AS, but the increase means teachers are gaining experience in teaching them. And you may just find a Godsend of a teacher who wants more reading – or is interested in attending seminars or conferences on AS as part of their continuing education training.

It also helps if your child can have a school "safe harbor." This could be a counselor or other person at the school that your child can seek out if he or she becomes overwhelmed and needs an understanding soul to help put things back on track. Setting up this safe harbor before the school year starts – and helping your child understand when and how to go to this person -- can be a lifesaver.

From the time our son was diagnosed with Asperger Syndrome, we worked closely with his schools and sought out compatible teachers. There are a lot of great teachers out there and we were lucky to be able to help maneuver our son into some of their classrooms. An investment in skillful, tactful lobbying for the right teachers can make a tremendous difference in your child's school year.

A final thought. Especially in the younger grades, the teacher is often the person who can most influence whether a child with Asperger Syndrome is accepted by the rest of the class. Our son Drew (who has AS) had some very rough times in his K-12 journey. Kids with AS often are among the last ones picked for teams – and this hurts. But in one class, when the kids were picking academic teams, they would clamor that they wanted Drew on their side, because he always knew the answers. You can imagine what this did for his self-esteem.

Find a teacher who can help other children see and respect your child's strengths, and you've given your child and that teacher something they can hold onto not just for a year, but for the rest of their lives.

###

24 FIRST DAY OF SCHOOL SUCCESS TIPS

Most of us can remember some wonderful and terrible things about school. In many ways, the first day of class can set the tone for a whole school year. If you have a child with special needs, you can help lay the groundwork for a successful year's launch with some basic preparations.

Start by anticipating things from your child's point of view. What is he going to encounter and how is he likely to react?

Get in touch with school personnel and do some research.

- What will be your child's schedule?
- Who will his teachers be?
- What subjects will she take?
- What activities will he be involved in?
- How long will she spend at each activity?
- How will he need to physically move about the building during the day?

I'm a video producer. I can tell you from experience that one key to a successful day's shooting is scouting a location in advance.

You can use this same technique to help ensure a successful school year launch.

Contact your school staff before classes start and arrange a "preview" visit for you and your child. Get a staff member to explain what's going to happen on that first day step by step. Do a location walk-through with your guide, checking out hallways, classrooms, restrooms, cafeteria, gym, playground, sports fields — the works. Meet as many of the teachers and other school staff who your child will encounter that first day as possible. Discuss the schools rules. Find out what students should and shouldn't do. If he'll ride a school bus, get the details about pick-ups, drop-offs and the riding rules.

As you're touring, make some mental notes. Is your child interested or excited about anything in particular? Is there anything that he or she is likely to encounter that could trigger a sensitivity or problem behavior?

The more familiar your child becomes with the school, the staff, and what to expect, the better his chances of having a great first day. Knowing what will happen can also raise her confidence level and help her relate to other kids, as she'll be something of an expert on her surroundings.

After your visit, write out a one-page profile of your child for teachers and other staff. This should be a short outline or bullet points, and not a treatise. Note your child's strengths and challenges. Describe any difficult behaviors the school staff is likely to encounter and any effective ways you've found to deal with them. For example, you might note that your child sometimes becomes frustrated and angry in stressful situations, and that allowing him to go to a quiet corner of the room for a few minutes will usually enable him to calm down and rejoin class activities.

You're not using the document to tell teachers how to do their job. You're providing information to help them recognize what's happening from your child's point of view and use their best judgment to deal with the situation effectively.

It's best if you can use this profile as a guide for a pre-school year conference with your child's teachers. At the conference, you can hand out the profile, go into more detail about your child, and answer questions. Having the profile gives the teachers a resource they can refer to later, and helps lock what you've said in their memories. If possible, identify a staff member, such as a counselor, who your child can seek out if he or she gets stressed or has a problem. Your child should meet this person before school starts and know how to find or contact him or her during the school day.

The more teachers and other staff understand your child, the better they'll be able to respond appropriately to any quirks he or she may exhibit. I found a great example of this when I recently interviewed Karra Barber about her book, "Living Your Best Life With Asperger's Syndrome."

Kids with Asperger Syndrome tend to take things literally. Karra's son, Thomas, did just this when he got a call from a counselor at a camp he was about to attend. The counselors called the campers to introduce themselves and tell the kids what to expect at camp. Karra called her son to the phone, "Thomas...Tom, it's your counselor from camp!" When Thomas picked up the phone, the counselor (having heard his mom call him both Thomas and Tom) asked him what he'd like to be called.

"Ben," he said.

When Thomas and the counselor were finished talking, Karra confirmed with the counselor that her son's name was Thomas and they had a quick laugh.

After the call, Karra asked Thomas why he'd told the counselor to call him, "Ben."

He responded that the counselor had asked him what he'd like to be called and he told her "Ben" because he'd always liked that name.

It made complete sense from his point of view.

Giving teachers some insights into your child can help avoid misunderstandings and encourage them to use students' different perspectives to enrich their teaching. Giving your child a preview of his school can help prepare him for success.

You can think of a school year as a mountain road with a lot of twists and turns. A bit of preparation can serve as a guardrail to help your child and his teachers keep his car on the road, make good progress and enjoy the ride.

###

25 INNOVATION LIKE COLLABORATION

Have you ever had a great idea that turned out not so great? Or one that worked out, but only after you substantially tweaked it? Innovation is important, but often it needs to be tempered by collaboration to make sure it accomplishes its goal — without unwanted side effects.

Let me give you an example. A while back, someone got the idea to use a traffic light and alarm system in school cafeterias to help kids keep the noise level down. I learned about this product recently. I'm not sure when it was introduced, but I found a story about it in USA Today's Life section on October 12, 2004, titled: "Noise travels fast, but cafeteria ladies put a stop to it." A friend of our daughter who is in her 20's said she remembers having such a system in her elementary school cafeteria. So this system has been around for a while.

I found sites selling different versions of the product online, but it basically works like this: You put a traffic light, sensor, and alarm in your cafeteria. The traffic light glows green when things are relatively quiet. When student-generated noise builds to a preset level, the light changes to yellow and an alarm sounds. When the noise reaches a higher preset level, the light changes to red and a louder alarm sounds. Depending on the system, this louder alarm might be a buzzer, tone or siren. School officials can institute rules such as a five minute "no talking" ban after a red-light alarm.

Now, reducing cafeteria noise is a great goal. Our son, Drew, who has Asperger Syndrome, had real difficulty dealing with the noise levels in the cafeteria and at pep rallies while he was in middle school and high school. Loud noise levels overwhelm him and sudden loud noises startle him dramatically. Imagine someone unexpectedly shooting off a pistol next to your ear and you'll get an idea how loud noises (that wouldn't phase a person with average hearing) sound to Drew.

Of course, enforcing silence with alarms and sirens is more than a bit ironic. Especially when you consider the effect on children who are hypersensitive to loud noises. Not only can the alarm be painful, but anticipating the system going off can send these kids' anxiety levels through the roof. While school staff might install this system with the best of intentions, they may wind up with some children holding their ears in fear waiting for the audible assault — or trying to escape when a siren goes off and hurts their ears. It's happened.

This is just one "innovation" example. There are lots of ideas that may work well for most of a school population that can cause challenges for children with special needs; especially children with hypersensitivities or those who find changes in their routines threatening.

How can we help ensure that well-intended innovations work?

First, parents need to keep in close touch with school staff, make them aware of a child's sensitivities, and ask to be alerted to any changes in policies or practices that will affect students. It helps to recruit an advocate for your child who's on the staff. This could be a counselor, social worker or favorite teacher who knows your child's sensitivities. An advocate who is in a position to see potential problems can help find ways to avoid them, and, of course, keep parents in the loop so they can offer input. It helps if parents have frequent contact with this person or other school staff. Who knows what well-intentioned innovator in the school right now is planning something that could affect your son or daughter?

Second, schools need to carefully assess the impact of new policies and practices on individual students. Leaders need to share planned changes with staff and parents and ask for input on pros and cons. Networking can be invaluable for teachers planning significant changes in their classrooms that involve areas outside their experience. It's a rare policy, practice or system that covers all students' needs without some modifications or exceptions. Some children with special needs require extra preparation to deal with change. Some may need to be accommodated with an alternative activity. And, if an innovation that seemed like a great idea doesn't work, we all respect staff who are confident and flexible enough to either modify it or rescind it and move on to something else. Some of the best innovations involve an element of trial and error.

For Drew, the solution to his cafeteria sound sensitivities had some added benefits. Drew's middle school set up a social skills class for Drew and some other children over lunch once a week in a counselor's office. Then one of Drew's teachers volunteered to eat lunch with him on her break in her classroom on the other four days. So, Drew was able to eat his lunch in relative quiet, and he gained some weekly experience interacting with classmates. This alternative solved a significant problem caused by cafeteria noise. Eating away from the lunchroom would have been even more important if Drew's cafeteria had been equipped with a siren.

In high school, the staff allowed Drew to go to the library during pep rallies to avoid the loud noise.

Some of the best solutions are those you find by anticipating problems and avoiding them. If you're a parent, only you can determine how often you need to be in touch with school staff to accomplish this. However, if you have a child with special needs, I'd recommend having at least weekly contact. Daily contact is not too often in some cases. And beware of depending on your child to keep you up to speed. He or she may not know about planned changes, and some kids don't tell parents about difficulties even long after they've started.

Collaboration has historically been a friend to innovation.

A while back, former BCC science reporter James Burke produced a series on innovation called, "Connections." He made the point that the idea of the lone inventor toiling away and having a solitary "Eureka!" moment was often a myth. Many of the people we consider mankind's greatest inventors built on the work of others or collaborated with others or consulted with others to refine their ideas.

Collaboration helps us identify both the possibilities and pitfalls of our brainstorms and adjust accordingly to boost benefits and avoid mistakes we'd regret. Collaboration also helps parents and school staff develop consistent approaches so guidance and discipline at home and school reinforce each other.

We need innovation in our schools. Frequent parent-staff contact and lots of input on new ideas can help ensure we find and institute changes that work for students, staff and parents. And isn't that what we're all looking for?

###

26 APPRECIATING TEACHERS

I heard New York's 2007 teacher-of-the-year, Marguerite Izzo, on a PBS News Hour report the other day describe how she does "five shows daily." She appears to be a dynamo, who makes every lesson interesting.

It's no surprise that you need to be at least somewhat exciting and engaging in class to compete for kids' mindshare with videogames, cell phone cameras and text messaging.

Some teachers are born performers. Others have to learn to keep their students' attention. Either way, I think we need to appreciate all it takes to get up in front of a tough audience of modern school kids and try to reach into their complex, fast paced, media-tuned minds. And "performing" is only one aspect good teaching.

So, as the school year draws to a close, here's a thank you to the teachers we admire:

For understanding that the real measure of teaching is not what you cover, but what you can get your students to absorb.

For often putting your personal problems on hold and bringing your "A" game to class.

For igniting students' interest in things that matter.

For spending hours of work time outside the classroom that your students never see.

For constantly assessing and adjusting your approach, looking for the best ways to reach your students.

For not being afraid to try new techniques.

For working with parents to give students consistent messages and reinforcement at home and at school.

For accepting that students with physical or mental challenges are just as deserving of your time and attention as "typical" students.

For showing "difficult" students that you still believe in them when others have given up.

For thinking of every new class as "your" students.

For seeing students as individuals and seeking out their strengths.

For celebrating students' accomplishments.

For staying connected to students after they leave your class.

For knowing that if you can reach just one student in your class…but then, reaching just one student was never an option for you, was it?

For accepting students as they are, as you help them become what they can be.

Before I close, I'd like to go back to that News Hour report, by Time Magazine essayist Nancy Gibbs. It cited a National Education Association poll of teachers that asked what gift would make them feel most appreciated. The top response by a landslide? To hear someone say "Thank you."

Here's hoping that deserving teachers everywhere receive that reward.

###

27 EMPATHY IN THE CLASSROOM

Let me tell you about the worst "teacher" I ever had.

He was a salesman standing in for a trainer who'd gotten ill. He'd come to our company's location to teach a roomful of us to use a complicated, computer controlled, multi-projector slide show system. This salesman made a classic teaching mistake. He assumed that because something he worked with every day was easy for him to understand, it should be easy for others to pick up. He rattled off information about the system in machine-gun fashion. When he repeatedly asked us if we understood something and various class members said, "No," he impatiently snapped his fingers at us and barked, "Keep up, keep up!"

Some students got disgusted and left the class at the break. Others stuck it out, but learned little.

The salesman's failure was based on his inability to put himself in someone else's place, understand things from that person's point of view, and communicate information in a way, and at a pace, the person can absorb it.

Successful teachers either know these steps instinctively or learn them from experience.

Now it's time to throw you a curve. This article is not about teachers. It's about classmates of students who have Asperger Syndrome, High Functioning Autism or similar Autism Spectrum Disorders (ASDs).

Classmates can't be expected to have the instincts or experience of teachers. Many classmates are impatient with or dismissive of students who exhibit different or difficult behaviors due to ASDs, without ever knowing the reasons for those behaviors. It doesn't seem fair to simply get angry with these classmates, if they've never been given an explanation or been instructed how to interact with students who think and act differently.

There are no guarantees that educating students about ASDs is going to make all classmates more empathetic. But time after time, we've seen classmates who get that information become more understanding, accommodating and supportive. Especially if they're given the opportunity to mentally put themselves in the place of a student with an ASD and see things from his or her point of view. This helps them understand the reasons for impulsive behaviors, or seemingly tactless remarks, or sensitivities to light or sound or touch. Also, an important part of any such presentation is helping classmates become aware of students' strengths as well as their challenges.

And you don't have to single out a child on the spectrum or disclose a specific disability to hold a class lesson or school assembly about understanding students who think and act differently. While we've generally found that disclosing specific ASDs to classmates is helpful, that's a decision to be made by an individual student and his or her family.

If you're a teacher who has a student with an ASD in your class, consulting with parents and school staff and holding an education session about autism spectrum conditions can help integrate that student into your class and teach classmates valuable life lessons about tolerance, empathy and communication at the same time.

You don't want your students growing up to be the salesman who doesn't bother to read his audience and fails miserably to communicate.

Imagine your students looking back on your class gratefully as they succeed in business and life using the approach to understanding and reaching people that you've fostered.

As they enter an increasingly complex, multi-cultural, global workplace, yours could be a class they'll never forget. I hope someday you get letters, telling you just that.

###

28 TODAY IS GOING TO BE DIFFERENT

Matt's eyes dart around the classroom. Jennifer smiles shyly at him as their eyes meet. His pulse is racing. Everyone is getting seated and class is about to start.

Today is going to be different.

Yesterday, his class learned about Asperger Syndrome. The school counselor came and told everyone what it was and how it affected Matt. The counselor had talked with Matt and his parents beforehand, and they had agreed about what the counselor would say. He didn't make it sound like a disease or a big problem. Instead, the counselor explained that Matt's brain processed information differently in some ways, and that made some things harder for Matt. But he also described how it helped make Matt an expert at other things.

Matt looks up at the teacher and she smiles at him, too. The knot in Matt's stomach starts to undo itself. School had only begun a week ago, and it had started out to be as bad as last year.

Last year, Matt's teacher had never really understood what was going on in Matt's head. She'd gotten impatient when he continually forgot to raise his hand and called out answers in class. One terrible day, she'd accused him of not trying hard enough to control himself and asked him angrily if he knew what manners were. Overwhelmed by fear and confusion, he'd had a meltdown and started to cry. Then he'd had to walk, in shame, to the principal's office, where he'd gotten a lecture about acting his age. For the remainder of the year, some classmates had teased him and the rest had ignored him.

But now, his new teacher and the students around him knew there was a reason for the ways he acted and reacted.

Yesterday, the counselor had observed that everyone in the class was a bit different. He'd talked about looking past different behaviors to find the person underneath, pointing out that people like Wolfgang Amadeus Mozart, Sir Isaac Newton and Thomas Jefferson all had habits that made them look odd. This didn't mean that they had Asperger Syndrome or that anyone who acted different was a genius, but it did show what the world would have missed if people hadn't looked past their odd behaviors.

Then Matt had walked to the front of the room and talked about Asperger Syndrome and answered questions about it. Some of his classmates looked amazed when he described his love of sports statistics and easily answered their questions about their favorite teams and players. Matt felt like they were seeing him for the first time.

This morning, in the hall on his way to class, several kids had come up to Matt and apologized for the way they'd treated him. Jason had actually told two jerks from another class to lay off when they'd called Matt a retard.

Matt's mind comes back to the present as the teacher starts class. He knows he's still going to be seen as different. But now, maybe most of his classmates will be more patient and explain the social things he doesn't understand. He doesn't want to change everything about himself. He just wants to fit in. For the first time, that seems possible.

So this is what hope feels like.

(Matt's story is not about one child. It's a compilation with input from many stories I've heard from parents, teachers, and children. The last line is a quote from my son, who has Asperger Syndrome.)

###

Dan Coulter

DEALING WITH ASPERGER SYNDROME

29 DISCOVERING ASPERGER SYNDROME

Getting a diagnosis of Asperger Syndrome for your child is sort of like getting hit by a slow freight train. Usually, you know something's wrong. Maybe you got worried. Maybe teachers or others urged you to get your child checked out. Maybe, like my wife and I, you went through several other diagnoses first. But even though you knew something was coming, you still feel the impact when you get the official word.

I spoke with the parents of a newly diagnosed child recently. His mother said she had virtually shut down. She felt overwhelmed and almost paralyzed. She and her husband had demanding jobs. She knew how she'd planned her family's lives, but things were going to be so different...

Want the good news? You can make things get better. Sometimes amazingly better than may seem possible at first.

Don't get me wrong; Asperger Syndrome was one of the toughest things to happen to our family. But our 21 year-old son, Drew, who has Asperger Syndrome, was one of the best.

Drew is smart and funny and caring. He's also sometimes distracted and disorganized and overly sensitive. He's always tried hard to relate to people, but often lacked the tools and intuitive instruction manual to build friendships. Middle school and high school were especially tough. Academics went well, but interacting with pre-teen and teenage peers often seemed like trying to swim in storm-tossed waves while the water was calm for everyone else.

But he never gave up. During his last two years in high school, he finally starting making the kind of friendships he'd always wanted. Now he's in college. Toward the end of school breaks, he's eager to get back to the campus to be with his friends. And his life's getting better every year. It's light-years better than I could have imagined when we got his diagnosis.

If you've recently received a diagnosis of Asperger Syndrome for your child, here are some thoughts.

In your mind, separate your child from his challenges. Think of Asperger Syndrome as a tiger that has attached itself to your child for life. Your child is not the tiger, but you and your child both have to deal with the tiger. Sometimes you have to get past the tiger to reach your child. But, you can also find ways to make having a tiger work to your child's advantage.

You can make things better. Absolutely. No matter what your child's challenges, you can help improve things by finding and reinforcing his strengths – and by helping him overcome his weaknesses. Spending time with a child having fun is one of the best gifts ever. When you're a child, seeing your worth in your mother or father's eyes can give you strength to last a lifetime and the courage to never give up.

People with AS often describe themselves as looking at the world in a different way. Give your child the benefit of the doubt. Not everything he or she wants to do differently is a problem that needs to be fixed. It may just be another way to reach the same goal. And he may have special abilities that can help him excel in the right job.

Patience pays off. Expect results, but not always quick results. It took my son years to learn to manage social interactions and to make friends. Years. But all the social skills coaching and positive reinforcement were worth it. Also, one of the secrets is to get your child together with kids who have similar interests. My son, for example, loves Japanese "anime" animation, and that's helped him connect with a number of friends. Drew feels his life now is dramatically better than it was in high school.

Social skills are golden. Common, everyday, social interaction is the most universal challenge for kids with AS. Helping your child learn about the give and take of dealing with people can make a huge difference in how others treat him and how he sees himself. Some kids practice the piano. If your child spends that same kind of time practicing social skills, you'll never regret it.

Don't underestimate your son or daughter. It's easy to give your child a lifetime handicap by assuming he or she can't do this or that. Most kids with AS can learn to compensate to some extent for things that don't come naturally. Set high goals and help your child master independent life skills along the way. It's hard to learn to fly if you never get the chance to solo.

Beware perfectionism. Mastering a skill doesn't always mean perfecting it. Sometimes "good enough" really is good enough. Your child may make A's in school, but it may take even more effort for him to make a C or B in "eye contact" or "listening without interrupting" or other social skills. If your child is really trying and making progress, not pushing too hard for perfection can save everyone a lot of stress. And praise is a great lubricant to success. Criticism can be like sand in the gears.

Finally, look at your opportunities. You don't want your child to have problems, but helping him or her deal with those problems can bring you closer. You don't have to thank a storm for helping you get to know your shipmates – but you can be grateful for their friendship just the same. Working with your child can help you form a bond that you might otherwise have missed.

Plenty of people without Asperger Syndrome have it rough. When I think of the problems my son has never had -- drinking, drugs, violence, crime -- I feel pretty lucky. As a family, we've had lots of experiences that make me grin every time I think of them. We have fun whenever we're together. Life is only as special as you make it.

Drew's life will surely be different. It will sometimes be tough. But, with our support, he's making it full, rich and meaningful.

Tiger and all.

###

30 ASPERGER SYNDROME: DIFFERENCE OR DISABILITY?

Is Asperger Syndrome a difference or a disability? I've read a lot about this question and seen people come down strongly one way or the other. With my son, who has AS, newly home from college and starting a job search, I've had an opportunity to take a fresh look at the whole issue.

At college, Drew lived in a dorm, managed his own schedule, succeeded academically and made a circle of friends. His graduation was a tremendous accomplishment.

But finish lines are often also starting lines for the next event. And you may need more and different skills for the new contest. Having Drew live at home again and interact with us on a daily basis helped me realize that his college was a more flexible and accepting environment than many workplaces may be.

Workplaces can be very competitive and have their own cultures and rules. With all he learned and accomplished, Drew's college experience didn't erase his Asperger Syndrome. I thought about this as our family sat in a theater recently before a movie. Drew made a comment to me, his mother and sister, but in a voice loud enough to be heard by several rows of audience members.

This made me think about how often social skills are as important as task skills in a workplace. I started mentally listing some areas -- some fairly subtle -- that I wanted to work on with Drew to help him improve his prospects of getting and keeping a job.

But then, I thought, how far should I take this? The comment Drew made was a bit too loud for the social setting, but it was also witty and funny. Asperger Syndrome can create behaviors that put people at a disadvantage and "disable" them in some ways. But if we push too hard to modify the "disablers," we risk disabling some of the strengths and personality traits that make them who they are.

A few days ago, Drew drove off to be with a group he found that hangs out at a book store on Friday nights. "It's just really great to be with people who accept me for who I am," he said before he left.

I want to help my son refine his social skills to get and hold a job, and I also want him to see me as someone who accepts him for who he is.

Like most things in life, it's a balancing act. If we see AS solely as a either a disability or a difference, we risk smothering a unique personality or not giving help where it's truly needed.

As we counsel and advise our kids (and we are, of course, going to counsel and advise them), we need to make sure we don't push so hard in so many areas that we discourage them and sabotage our efforts. We need to pick out things that will really make a difference and help our sons and daughters see the benefits of making those changes. And we need to let go of the stuff that's not as crucial.

I don't ever want to change the core things that make Drew, Drew.

Talking too loud is not the biggest problem you can have — especially when you have something to say.

###

31 DIFFERENT MEANS DIFFERENT

Most of us tend to judge people by how they compare to us. When we run into someone completely different, we usually try and fit him into the framework of our past experience.

Someone who can't do something we can do, especially after we've shown him how to do it or he's done it before, may seem slow or stubborn or just not trying hard enough.

But sometimes, different means different, and there's nothing in our experience that prepares us to deal with him. I'm thinking primarily of kids who have Asperger Syndrome or a similar diagnosis on the autism spectrum.

My son has Asperger Syndrome (AS) and I've been interacting with him for 23 years now. He's accomplished a tremendous amount and I'm enormously proud of him, but sometimes his approach to things baffles me.

It really helps to remind myself that he sees and reacts to some things differently than almost everyone else. And that's part of the challenge. Even when I know he has AS, he's so smart and funny and insightful about so many things, it can still take me off guard when he doesn't automatically do something I assumed he would see as important.

At these times, recalling that he truly has a different perspective helps prevent me from kicking into "Frustration Mode." In Frustration Mode, our brains and adrenal glands insist on a quick fix. We can harden our voices and demand things of our kids that don't work and only make the situation worse.

The problem can be even more difficult when our kids encounter teachers or others who find our kids not just different, but new to them and extremely different.

I recently read something a mother had written about her teenage son finally being able to explain what had been going on with him for years. Sometimes a teacher would call on him and he'd know the answer, but be unable to voice it. At other times his mind would go blank. But this only happened intermittently.

Picture being seen as a bright kid who's unmotivated or stubborn or a smart aleck. Think of trying to please a teacher or parent and having him respond with disappointment or disapproval or discipline. Imagine sometimes being trapped in your own head.

Even if we know our kids have challenges, it's easy to forget that these challenges don't always appear consistently or in the same manner. It's also sometimes hard to remember that we may not know everything about how autism affects our kids. It's crucial to keep an open mind and keep an extra batch of patience in our back pockets. Some parents do this and seem to also have an "auxiliary patience backpack" at their disposal. I really admire these parents.

I'm not saying we shouldn't be firm and discipline our kids when they need it. But calm, firm discipline that gives our kids the benefit of the doubt is a much different approach than launching into Frustration Mode. If you find yourself in Frustration Mode, it's best to delay issuing any edicts until you can calm down and think things through.

And while we're working on our own skills, it's important to make sure that teachers, coaches, and anyone else who's going to have significant responsibility for our kids understand how their brains can work differently. It's also helpful to explain what is and isn't effective in dealing with an individual child.

I spoke with a mother the other day who went on a study trip with her high school-aged son, who has Asperger Syndrome. She and her son didn't disclose to the other people on the study trip, sponsored by a college, because her son is bright and could do the work, and his mother was along to smooth the social issues. This worked out fine for them. However, there was another student along on the trip who the mother quickly assessed was on the autism spectrum. The trip leaders couldn't figure out what caused the student's different behaviors and, according to the mother, didn't handle the situation well. This mother had a private talk with the leaders to make them aware of the probable reasons for the student's behaviors, but overall, it was a wrenching experience for the student.

We need to be confident that other adults know how to deal with our kids before we put our kids in their care. Volunteering to accompany your child's group during an activity or trip is often a good alternative.

For parents of newly diagnosed children, I should admit that many of us veterans have succumbed to the temptation to send our kids into a situation where we suspected we should disclose a "difference," but didn't and hoped for the best. When and how to disclose is a personal decision based on each situation, but I urge you to weigh the pros and cons carefully as you're making these decisions.

When adults and peers notice the things about our kids that we hope they won't notice, their imaginations can come up with extreme explanations that can be way off the mark. Even when you disclose, information doesn't automatically inject competence and compassion into people who are prejudiced and close-minded. But in my experience, our kids are usually treated better -- often much better -- if people know the reasons for their different behaviors.

This is about letting go of what might have been and making things as good as they can be in the real world. It's sometimes amazing how accepting and supportive people can be -- and how our kids tend to blossom, enjoy life and achieve when they're accepted for who they are.

After I'd been a father for a few years, a co-worker expecting her first child asked me about becoming a parent. I said, "It's more wonderful and terrifying than you can possibly imagine." I still think that's true. But the more you grab reality and run with it, the more you can temper the terror. As for the wonderful parts, you find they're largely up to you, and absolutely worth the ride.

###

Dan Coulter

32 DEALING WITH KIDS' SETBACKS

Some days it just seems all too much. You get a call from the school about an incident with your son. Or your daughter comes home defiant and tearful. And whatever you do seems like the wrong thing.

Well, it's probably not. The right thing to do isn't always the perfect thing. Or rather, you don't need to find the perfect solution to do something that helps. If you're like most parents (and by most parents, I mean, me) you don't routinely hit the ball out of the park. There's a fair amount of trial and error involved.

And it's even more of a challenge as your child gets older. We usually do too much or too little. But it helps when you start to understand that this is the way it works. Raising children, and especially children with special needs, is a constant state of discovering what - and how much -- to do. For one thing, you never know how much independence they can handle until you give them too much.

It's sort of like being in a sailboat. Whatever your destination, you're constantly dealing with winds trying to blow you off course. You often have to tack back and forth, not always able to steer exactly toward your goal, but constantly getting closer, until you reach it.

Just as we can't usually sail directly to our goals, we often can't help our kids solve problems immediately. But if we keep providing course corrections and don't get discouraged, we can help them make steady progress.

Of course, sometimes it's hard not to get discouraged. And sometimes we're too close to an event to see the better courses of action. So we need to be careful about making decisions affecting the future in a fury of frustration. "We're never going to a fast food restaurant again!" or "I'm going to call that child's mother and give her a piece of my mind!" Radical solutions can sometimes do more harm than good.

Better to wait and look at the problem with the perspective a little time can give, even if it's only an hour or a day. And it always helps to step outside the problem and look at it objectively. What caused the problem? What can you or your child do differently?

If you need to convince your child to do something different, what incentives can you come up with? Focus on how he can get something he wants if he takes a certain course of action. And success is an amazing teacher. If a child tries something and it works, she'll almost always put it in her bag of tricks.

In my experience, negative consequences tend to shut down kids' minds. But even stubborn minds tend to seek out pleasure and the prospect of positive results. Be careful of getting dragged down into a contest of wills. "Because I say so," is not a convincing argument. And kids often find creative ways around obeying ultimatums. You've got to be the parent. You may not be smarter than your kids (I know this first-hand), but you have more experience. And you have a secret weapon. You love them even when they lose control.

They may be overwhelmed by the moment and frozen in injustice or disappointment or hopelessness. But adults tend to understand that there are few things more powerful than knowing someone cares about you and believes in you no matter what. Just listening to their frustration or anger can help defuse it. Have you ever seen your child so upset that he didn't want anyone suggesting solutions? You just don't UNDERSTAND! It's an insult to suggest there was anything else he could have done! It was just UNFAIR!

By staying calm, you can help the storm pass. You can be the safe haven. You can repair the torn sails and restock the ship and supply fresh navigation charts. And give your child the confidence to try again.

Belief is a powerful force. If you convince your daughter she can succeed, her chances of reaching a goal go up dramatically. Sometimes, belief is everything.

My wife has an uncle (Uncle William) who had a setback as a high school junior. When he got his report card at the year's end, it said he'd flunked -- and would have to repeat the 11th grade. William anxiously had a friend take the report card to his mother while he went to his after-school job delivering telegrams. When he got home, he found his mother had fixed him his favorite dinner, fried chicken, and baked him a big apple pie. And she didn't say a word about his report card that night. The next day, they sat down together and came up with a plan.

In spite of being scared, William went alone to the school and negotiated an agreement that he could go on to the 12th grade with his class if he retook some key courses in summer school and passed. He did just that. And he went on to succeed in college and graduate school. Today, Uncle William is a respected minister and community leader.

Love and understanding can see you through the toughest times and give your kids a lifelong example to follow.

So, the next time your child has a setback, you have an opportunity. You can understand that setbacks are not an interruption of the process; they're part of the process. However you decide to help, it can be the right thing even if it's not the perfect thing.

And you can't go wrong with apple pie.

###

33 KIDS NEED EACH OTHER

I think kids need each other.

Kids don't just learn from parents and teachers, they learn from other kids. One of the most important lessons they can learn is how to get along with people who don't look or think or act exactly like they do.

That's why I believe everyone -- typical kids, gifted kids, and kids with special needs – should be interacting in schools. That doesn't mean I'm opposed to advanced placement classes or self-contained classrooms for special needs kids. I'm in favor of these kinds of groupings, as long as they're really designed as the best way to teach the students involved and are not an excuse to isolate kids from each other.

Whenever it's practical, I think it's good to have kids with special needs in mainstream classes with other kids -- and to have schools actively support positive interactions between kids of all ability levels in and out of class. Active support is crucial here. Special needs kids interacting with typically developing classmates without adequate supervision and support can get eaten alive.

It's especially important to integrate kids who don't look or act quite like everyone else.

There are a range of conditions such as Asperger Syndrome, Higher Functioning Autism, Pervasive Developmental Delay, Semantic-Pragmatic Disorder (the list goes on and on), that can make kids appear different to their classmates. Many of these kids have normal to superior intelligence and can do the academic work that's required in regular or advanced classes.

Their differences, however, can serve as a wall between them and their peers. Maybe one has a processing problem that makes his speech slow, a second is sensitive to loud noises and a third has a hard time making conversation. If the other kids in the class avoid these kids because of their differences, they may never find out that one is an expert on fish, another is an astronomy prodigy and a third can do complex math problems in her head. Or, the "different" kids may just have similar interests to their classmates.

While these artificial walls isolate kids who are different, they also diminish the other kids in the class. Not only do they miss out on knowing some interesting classmates, they risk forming a habit of only seeking out and associating with people who look and act like themselves.

Countries are becoming more culturally diverse. National economies have largely merged into a global economy. Kids who learn to investigate differences and interact with a variety of people will have a tremendous advantage when they leave school and enter the real world – and kids who don't will be at a disadvantage.

When we judge people only by their differences and don't look any deeper, it's easy to make false assumptions or to miss opportunities.

I got a lesson about making assumptions when I worked in the corporate world. In a team-building exercise, I was with a group of co-workers given a challenge to cross a pretend river. Standing in a field, we were given some wooden two-by-fours to make a narrow bridge. As a team, we had to figure out how to lay the boards across some rocks so we could all cross the "river" without stepping off the boards. There were some other conditions that made it a brain teaser to lay out the boards and get us all across inside the allowed time limit. To make it more interesting, one of our group had a bandana placed over her eyes and was labeled, "blind."

We gamely took on the project and managed to get everyone across the river. That was when the folks running the exercise evaluated how we'd treated our blind colleague. While we had carefully guided her over the boards, we hadn't once asked her advice or tried to include her in our planning. We'd seen her only as a liability. Suppose the "blind" person was actually the smartest and most inventive in the group? What if she'd been an engineer? We'd ignored her possible contributions because we hadn't even tried to look past her disability.

It's easy for most of a student body to do the same thing with kids in "special ed" or kids in regular classes who are a bit different. Whatever these kids' capabilities or challenges, classmates will never know what they might contribute if we don't actively encourage kids of all stripes to interact in positive ways. That's why schools need programs and materials to educate all students to look past differences and see reasons to connect.

These sorts of connections can help every kid. They can help students with serious disabilities learn to deal with others and be as self-sufficient as possible, making more of them employable and fewer of them candidates for public assistance. They can help typical and non-typical students see each others' strengths. They can help gifted students see the benefits of sharing their gifts unselfishly. And they can encourage an entire student body to become the enlightened, compassionate people whom we want running the world in the next generation.

I've seen this kind of culture in a number of schools. I'd love to see us commit to develop it in all our schools. The widespread creation of school anti-bullying programs is a big step in the right direction.

Academics are important, but helping kids learn to reach out to each other as human beings can be the glue that holds us together as the world gets more complex.

Our kids need more than degrees. Our kids need each other.

###

34 WHERE'S THE MANUAL?

If your child is diagnosed with a significant disability, disorder or condition, it's pretty common to start a frantic search for answers. Is there a cure? If there's no cure, where's the manual I can use to do exactly the right things to help my child make his life as good as it can possibly be?

How do I deal with his behaviors? Can I help him change them? Should I? Should she be medicated? Should she go to public or private school? What kind of doctor should he see? What should I tell her siblings? Can I help him learn to support himself when he grows up? What should I do about this and this and this?

My wife, Julie, and I went through this process with our son, Drew, who has Asperger Syndrome (AS). AS is a neurobiological condition on the higher functioning end of the autism spectrum.

The good news is, our 24 year old son is doing fine and we've had big fun with him and his 23 year old sister, Jessie, as they've grown up. Of course, we also had tough times. Some of the toughest were dealing with the unknowns. But the more we learned about our kids and their conditions -- and found ways to make their lives better and their futures brighter -- the better we felt.

There's nothing that gives you a charge like helping your child master a skill or conquer a problem, especially if it helps put your mind at ease about his future. And whatever a child's challenges, a caring, determined parent (or two) can make a dramatic difference in her prospects for the future.

Thinking back on raising our kids, I thought I'd share some of the things that helped us.

GET MOVING

Start your search for answers quickly. Even when you can't see the end of the road, or know exactly where it will lead you, it helps to know you're moving in the direction of helping your child. For example, early in our journey we heard a good piece of advice: treat your son or daughter with a condition as a child first and a patient second. Parents tend to treat kids differently if they see them primarily as patients. Julie also attended educational conferences whenever possible to learn more about AS.

NETWORK, NETWORK, NETWORK

Talk to professionals, foundations, support groups and gather as much information as possible from materials related to your child's diagnosis. If you don't have a diagnosis or aren't sure you've got the right diagnosis, search for information about your child's symptoms or behaviors. Drew had seven successive diagnoses before we got one that fit like a glove: Asperger Syndrome. Looking back, it appears now that some of these diagnoses were influenced with the specialty of the doctor making them. For example, a psychologist diagnosed "personality disorder." Of course, many of these diagnoses came before Asperger Syndrome was included in the U.S. Diagnostic and Statistical Manual. Some of the best information we got came late in this process from a developmental pediatrician, who had experience with children like Drew. If we'd known that such a specialty existed at the beginning of our search, we could have honed in on a more accurate diagnosis more quickly.

TRUST YOURSELF

You may see a battalion of specialists, but none of them will spend as much time with your child as you do. Write down your concerns, observations and questions before a doctor visit so you can be sure you won't forget anything. If a professional's diagnosis doesn't match what you see in your child or their treatments don't help, let them know. If a professional doesn't take your concerns seriously or doesn't explain things to your satisfaction, it's appropriate to search for someone who does.

I am NOT saying that you should diagnose your child yourself and shop doctors until you find one who agrees. I am saying you should find a doctor or other professional who really listens to you and is willing to consider your input seriously -- and one who can explain his diagnosis and recommended treatment in a way that makes sense to you.

GET ANGRY, GET DISCOURAGED, GET OVER IT, MOVE ON

In dealing with conditions such as AS, there are times when you feel angry, frustrated or overwhelmed, that you just don't know enough to make the right decisions. If you find yourself feeling like that, remember that you're not in this alone. There are professionals and support groups and other resources available and you can learn a lot from them. You're also going to be learning more about your child every day. You can't gauge how well you're going to do by what you know at the beginning of the process. It's bit like having a baby for the first time. Some of it will be trial and error and everyone makes a few mistakes, but you'll learn more and more of the answers and become more confident as time goes by. As for doctors, you can find a gem the first time out, but if you don't, keep looking.

BECOME AN EXPERT ON YOUR CHILD'S SCHOOL

School was a joy for our daughter, Jessie. Less so for Drew. A preschool teacher saw his problems interacting with other kids and suggested we have him tested. At first we resisted. He was such a bright little guy, how could there be anything wrong? But then we saw her point and began our search for the right diagnosis and treatment. During most of Drew's early grade school years, we lived in a county with an exploding population — and a school district struggling to build schools and hire teachers fast enough to keep up. They simply didn't have programs to support children like Drew, who got good grades but had trouble connecting with other kids. It wasn't that the school administrators were bad-intentioned or negligent, but they were busy putting out fires. Our son was smoldering, but he wasn't on fire. We were ready to start a search for a good private school when we moved to another part of the country and found a public school district with the staff and resources to really help a kid like Drew. Through a series of diagnoses, he got support based on his needs, even before his diagnosis of Asperger Syndrome at age 14.

But it wasn't just that the school district was good. Julie got to know the teachers and administrators. She provided information to the school and served as a parent volunteer in a number of ways — including ways not directly related to our son. She found that establishing relationships with the school staff helped her become part of a team that took both Drew's needs and the needs of the school into account. This was often a key to working around obstacles.

As a part of this process, Julie enlisted a number of angels in the school. Angels are teachers or counselors or administrators who take a special interest in your child. Someone who will look out for him and who he knows he can go to when things get rough. Drew's about to graduate from college and we take great delight in regularly getting in touch with these angels and giving them credit for all they did to help him succeed.

Julie also kept great notes of her interactions with the school, including Individual Education Plan meetings and other contacts. Keeping accurate records helps when things are going well – and especially when they're not. For example, if you should find yourself in a school district where your child is not getting proper support, good documentation can help you work to correct the situation. It's our experience that it's always best to be as positive as possible when working with a school. Offering to serve as a resource rather than appearing to tell someone how to do his or her job has been a successful approach for us.

Also, frequent contact with teachers and staff helps you determine whether supports put in place to help your child are actually being delivered. If your child is supposed to get speech therapy twice a week and it stops for some reason, you want to know immediately, not at the end of the year.

When your child is not getting what the school agreed to or what the law requires, you many want to seek help from a parent advocate of a special needs support group. For example, here in North Carolina, the TEACCH program provides parent advocates where children on the autism spectrum are involved. Another good resource to consult about your child's rights is www.wrightslaw.com.

If you're moving, thoroughly check out the potential schools your child will attend and make them a significant factor in deciding where to buy a house.

KEEP YOUR EARS OPEN

Support groups, friends and Internet bulletin boards can all be great sources of advice. We've benefited from all three throughout the years. But we've also learned to check out informal advice with a critical eye. People's opinions are based on their experience, and their situations may be far different from yours. For example, we love the expression, "If you've seen one kid with Asperger Syndrome, you've seen one kid with Asperger Syndrome."

So we recommend that you keep your ears open. Listen to everyone, then do what makes sense to you. The more time you spend with your child and the more you learn, the better your radar will tell you who has good insights. The bottom line here is that whatever is diagnosed or prescribed or recommended by others, you as a parent have ultimate responsibility for making decisions for your child. The better informed you make yourself, the better decisions you can make.

BE POSITIVE

Many kids with disabilities face a lot of rejection. Having their home life be a haven of good feelings can be an important self-esteem safety net. And while I wouldn't wish a disability on anyone, you can find positive things in almost any situation. For example, dealing with our kids' challenges has brought us closer as a family. Also, if your child hears you complaining, you may make him an inadvertent messenger. Consider the consequences of having your child say to a teacher or principal, "My mom and dad say that you're _____." (Fill in the blank with some unkind thoughts you've had about someone.) Being positive and encouraging around your child can help him become a problem solver throughout his life.

TAKE CARE OF YOURSELF

We've learned you can take better care of your child if you take care of yourself. Finding some time for yourself -- and couples finding time to be together -- helps you come up with solutions to problems that seem insurmountable when you're stressed. If you think you don't have time to relax or you feel guilty taking time for yourself, do it because it will help you help your child. Really.

EDUCATE YOUR CHILD -- AND THE WORLD

One of my favorite themes is that raising a child with special needs is a 50-50 proposition. You need to prepare your child to deal with the world, but you also often may need to educate the world about your child. You can teach your child to modify some odd behaviors, but that won't help him make friends if classmates avoid him because they don't know why he struggles to make conversation. Disclosing a disability is and should be a personal choice for a child and his family. With that in mind, we've found that kids are often willing to befriend a classmate who's different if you just share a bit about why he acts like he does. Helping classmates, potential employers and others understand the reasons behind some of your child's behaviors can sometimes make the difference between rejection and acceptance.

IN CONCLUSION

These are some of the things we've learned along the road. Drew will receive his bachelor's degree in May and has already started his job search. He surprised us during college by starting a novel with a first chapter that impressed me as a writer. Jessie has a double major in music and international relations and recently returned from a two-week seminar studying government in Washington, D.C.

Sure, we worried a lot about doing the right things for our kids as they were growing up. But if you're like us, you'll find at some point that you have the manual you wanted.

You just have to write it yourself.

###

35 KIDS COUNT ON CONSISTENCY

If you're a parent or a teacher, can your kids or students count on you? I mean, do you think about being consistent so they know what to expect?

Kids who have Autism Spectrum Disorders, in particular, often benefit from guidance that's structured and consistent.

If a child has a habit that you want to modify, or needs to learn a skill, consistently reinforcing a behavior can help make it a part of that child's repertoire.

Try looking at the teaching process from his or her point of view. If we allow poor table manners at home, but try to enforce proper manners in a restaurant, we're sending mixed messages. It's much more practical for kids to learn one set of manners that's appropriate for both situations.

The world can seem chaotic to kids with ASDs. Think of them as pilots trying to land their planes. It's hard enough to land on a stable runway on the ground. But navy pilots will tell you it's a lot harder to land on an aircraft carrier deck that's heaving on the waves. As much as possible, we need to be the stable runways that our kids can depend on -- and consistently guide them toward behaviors that will be appropriate in the majority of situations they'll encounter.

I read something the other day written by a teacher who described a challenge with a former student who was on the autism spectrum. This student would sometimes express affection in ways that were inappropriate for a regular school classroom. The teacher gently redirected him toward other, more appropriate behaviors. However, some of his other teachers found his affectionate behaviors cute and encouraged them. The behaviors continued and caused the student increasing problems with teasing as he entered middle school.

This writer urged other teachers to guide their students' behaviors in light of the student's best interests, and to be consistent.

In Scotland County, North Carolina, they're restructuring a local high school of 1800 students into nine smaller, semiautonomous learning academies or "schools within a school." To ensure that Scotland High's programs are consistent with the needs of the real world, six advisory boards with business, community and teacher representatives are working together to establish the academies.

Each academy will have its own guidance counselor and every student will be assigned an adult advocate who'll stay with him until he graduates. Teachers within an academy will meet weekly to consult about the students they have in common. So instead of seeing a student only in light of the subject they teach, instructors will get a sort of "360 degree view" of each student. They can then develop coordinated, consistent teaching approaches based on an individual student's needs.

While we can't look to all our schools to restructure on this model, having parents and teachers find ways to bring a student's teachers together to consult frequently is a goal worth pursuing.

My son, Drew, who has Asperger Syndrome, had an instructional aide in high school. His aide mentioned how helpful it was to meet frequently with Drew's English teacher and an in-class support special education teacher. They'd compare notes and discuss teaching strategies so they could be consistent in helping Drew. School staff also set up a system to get feedback from Drew. Every Friday, Drew would meet with his school case manager and his aide for a "week in review" session. They'd discuss Drew's performance, encourage his progress and set goals for the coming week.

Speaking of feedback, we can sometimes throw up roadblocks to getting good input from our kids without meaning to. Have you ever asked a child about something he did and listened attentively if you liked the answer — but, if you didn't like his answer, interrupted him to criticize him and tell him what he should have done differently? Most of us have. Tends to shut off the information flow, doesn't it?

Being consistent in listening to answers we do and don't like can be a more effective approach. If you can steel yourself to ask questions and listen during your "research" conversations, then consider your approach and calmly offer your guidance a bit later, you may find you can collect more accurate information to work from.

Using this feedback, along with other input, you can determine a child's greatest needs and come up with a plan with consistent actions you can take to help him learn key skills or modify his behaviors.

Here's another thought on feedback from kids. If you don't get satisfying answers to your questions, it could have to do with how the child's brain processes information. If he hasn't thought about a subject, pressing him for an answer may cause him to clam up, or agree with something you're suggesting just to end a conversation that's stressful for him.

You may want to try telling him today to think about a subject that you'd like to discuss tomorrow. If tomorrow comes and he still can't tell you, say, what classes he'd like to take next year, you may want to offer him some choices, explain some of the options, and come back to the subject in another day. It may take a series of consistently calm conversations to help him consider what you're asking and give you useful input. This can also help him learn about the process of considering alternatives and making decisions.

Consistency in discipline is also an effective learning tool.

Some of us, parents and teachers, have problems modulating our discipline when we're in a "mood." If the same behavior in a child draws a sharp reprimand when we're tired and stressed, and no comment when we're calm and relaxed, we're not basing our guidance on what's best for our child or student.

Think of the ways being consistent helps us in society. Traffic laws say we have to signal before we make a turn, whether there's anyone in sight or not. If we get into the habit of signaling only when we see other drivers, we risk not noticing someone, not signaling and causing an accident. That's why the law tells us to signal consistently.

Think kids need to experience some inconsistency so they can learn how to deal with it? Don't worry, there's plenty of inconsistency built into daily life. There's no way to avoid it. But offering consistency where we can, like always putting daily homework assignments in the same place on a chalkboard or whiteboard, can be a real benefit for students. As a backup, you might place homework assignments on a website where students know they can always access them. Steps like these also can help show students the value of being consistent in their own lives.

Being consistent doesn't mean being inflexible. I think the best combination is to be consistent in offering guidance to our kids, but flexible in adapting to their needs. And there should always be room for creativity, spontaneity and fun in any plan you draw up. Consistency should be a launching pad for creativity, not a weight holding it down.

Ralph Waldo Emerson often gets misquoted as saying, "Consistency is the hobgoblin of little minds." What he actually said was, "A foolish consistency is the hobgoblin of little minds."

###

Dan Coulter

36 LEARNING SELF-ADVOCACY SKILLS

What's the most important skill a high school student with Asperger Syndrome or autism can learn before he or she graduates?

Run a list of candidate skills through your head. It's a good exercise.

Was self-advocacy on your short list? I think I can make a good case that it should be.

Whether your student is bound for a job or for college after graduation, he's almost certainly entering a much less protected environment. Many students on the autism spectrum are used to having a lot of things done for them. A student who hasn't learned to speak up for herself in high school isn't going to magically acquire the ability when handed a high school diploma.

If your son gets a job, will he ask the right questions if his boss gives him a task he doesn't understand?

If your daughter goes to college, how will she react if she doesn't catch the details of an assignment?

For many people on the spectrum, it's especially hard to speak up and ask for directions or for help. Sometimes that's because they don't want to call attention to themselves -- or look different. And many kids on the spectrum would be at a loss to explain their challenges and what accommodations they need to perform well in a job or in a college class.

At a recent admissions seminar at High Point University near my home, a counselor explained a common reason that students with disabilities appeared before the academic review board after receiving poor grades. It was almost always the case that the students either hadn't asked for accommodations, or hadn't used the accommodations that they had been granted.

I've heard a number of accounts where someone on the autism spectrum lost a job because of problems that started with miscommunication with a supervisor.

Knowing this, you can help your kids avoid these pitfalls. Your son or daughter doesn't have to disclose his or her condition to everyone, but when they need and want to, can they — and will they? By the way, it's common for parents to assume that a child on the spectrum knows more about his condition than he actually does.

So, find out what your student knows. Sit down with your son or daughter and talk about the importance of self-advocacy. Ask them what they know about their condition and about any accommodations they're receiving at school. Use what you discover to fill in any gaps in their knowledge, then plan a program of activities that will continuously build their ability to explain their condition without embarrassment and describe what they need in a particular situation. Sometimes, what they need may turn out only to be detailed instructions on how an assignment or job needs to be done.

Show them the benefits of learning self-advocacy by tying their progress to privileges. The more situations they show you they can handle, the more independence you give them.

If your child has an Individualized Education Program at his school, make sure he knows what's in it. Discuss the plan with him before school IEP meetings and help him take an active part in the meetings. Consider making one of your child's IEP goals that he develops the ability to explain his condition and describe his needed accommodations to an employer or instructor. If you need help with your IEP, there's an excellent article titled, "Writing Individualized Education Programs (IEPs) for Success" by Barbara D. Bateman on the "www.wrightslaw.com" website at this webpage: http://www.wrightslaw.com/advoc/articles/iep.success.bateman.htm

When your child has doctor appointments, get her used to talking to the doctor directly. You may want to explain to the doctor ahead of time, or at the beginning of the visit, that you're preparing your student to manage her own medical care, and that you'll be mainly an observer in the examining room.

It's also important to develop your child's ability to explain what he needs or wants when no mention of his condition is required. In stores, in restaurants, at events, etc., take every opportunity to have your student take the lead in interacting with people. Explain what he'll need to do in detail beforehand. You can stand by in case you're needed, but don't be too quick to step in and take over when there's a problem. You can think of yourself as a lifeguard. You don't want to let your charges drown, but everyone swallows a little water while learning to swim.

Recently, I interviewed Dorothy Wells, Assistant Director of Disability Support Services at the University of North Carolina at Pembroke. I asked her the most important things a high school student with Asperger Syndrome or autism should do to prepare for college. She said, "It's simple, start going to your IEP meetings and get comfortable talking to people about your special need."

You can think of self advocacy as a crucial "enabling skill" that allows your son or daughter to apply the other skills they've learned to succeed in class, in a career and in life.

Self-advocacy may not be the most important skill on your list of things to teach your high school student. But it may be the most important skill that's not on your list – and should be.

37 GET REAL

Will next year be better for you and your kids with special needs? "Gosh, I hope so," I hear you say. Me too. I want things to get better every year.

With two kids who have special needs, some years have been tough for our family. Recently, even with new challenges, things have been pretty darn good.

One of our best tools to make things better is to "get real." You get real when you do a reality check, examine all your assumptions and make changes to your family's lives.

Now usually, someone telling you to face reality is trying to get you to accept a harsh truth you've been avoiding and deal with disappointment. I think that's why many of us can be reluctant to think about changing the way we do things.

I find a "get real" session has exactly the opposite effect. It helps you let go of things that aren't working and try new approaches that can trigger sought-after progress.

My 23 year-old son, Drew, has Asperger Syndrome. I'm still finding out things about him, learning more about how he thinks, and discovering better ways to relate to him.

I got an insight the other day when I was interviewing Brian King, a licensed clinical social worker who has Asperger Syndrome. Brian learned about his AS in the process of getting an AS diagnosis for one of his sons. Now he counsels people with AS and autism, along with their families, employers and others.

Brian said that after his diagnosis, he realized that he's not good at multi-tasking. For example, the people Brian worked with expected him to make eye-contact and do the traditional things that indicate the average person is paying attention during a conversation. But listening and making eye contact at the same time was exhausting for Brian. He found that he's more of a uni-tasker. Not forcing himself to process visual information while he's listening allows him to more easily focus on what people are saying. If the people he works with can change their assumptions and accept less frequent eye-contact, he doesn't have to expend lots of energy on something that's culturally expected, but not always essential. This enables him to work more comfortably and concentrate more efficiently.

Talking with Brian helped me see some of my son's behaviors in a fresh light. I know that it's sometimes hard for Drew to maintain eye contact.

But perhaps the solution isn't helping him train himself to always look at people during conversations.

Maybe it's helping him focus on making eye contact when it's really necessary, but also accepting that it's not always worth the considerable effort. Maybe he can sometimes explain to people that it helps him think to look away while holding a conversation.

When you write your new year's resolutions this year, maybe you could write down the assumptions you've made about your special needs child. Then you could talk about your list in a "get real" session with your son or daughter. Maybe your child is now old enough to understand and explain something he couldn't before. Maybe she can help you revise your assumptions and plan new approaches that help you get along better and provide even better support for her future.

And then, maybe you can use what you've learned to help others understand people with special needs in the new year.

As for me, I'm thinking 2007 would be a good year for an Asperger "get real" remake of the movie, "Casablanca." I've already got a start on the dialog for the new Bogey and Bergman characters.

"Here's looking at you kid...or not."

Have a real special new year.

###

38 MELTDOWNS AND THE BIG PICTURE

What do you do when your child does something inappropriate and has a meltdown while playing with other children? After the bottom falls out of your stomach, that is. It's easy to be caught up in the moment and scold your child for anti-social behavior or insist that he calm down.

But for many children, particularly if they have a condition such as Asperger Syndrome or autism, these may be the worst things we can do.

Scolding or making demands of a child who is upset and screaming or crying often just adds fuel to an emotional fire. This can create an "overload loop" that keeps replaying in his or her mind.

Let's say you and two other parents are supervising your kids at a park where you arranged a play date — and your child falls apart.

You may be able to salvage the situation by breaking your child's train of thought. First, remove him from the immediate area and talk with him in a soothing voice until he calms down. Depending on his age, you may be able to distract him with a favorite toy or by encouraging him to talk about a special interest. Once he's in a more reasonable frame of mind, you can describe what he needs to do rejoin his playmates. Be clear about the advantages of doing what you ask. You may want to offer a reward if he's able to play according to the rules you give him.

But what if this approach doesn't work? We all want to fix problems quickly, but that's not always possible. Sometimes your best option may be to remove your child from the scene in a strategic retreat. It's important to see this as part of a strategy, not as a failure. You have to look at the big picture. Your short-term goal of a good play session may be foiled, but you can use what you learned to help accomplish your long-term goal of teaching your child to socialize with other children. Focusing on failure is a dead end. Concentrating on future success will help your child more.

Disclosure can be your ally. It's usually best to tell the other parents involved why your child acts the way he does and give them an opportunity to help. Not disclosing may actually drive them away, if they just see a case of kids not getting along. Playmates may not need to know about a specific diagnosis, but if their parents explain what behaviors they're likely to see, and suggest what to do when they occur, they're more likely to be accommodating. And disclosing a specific condition to other children when they're old enough to understand is usually a good idea.

Consider ways to structure play sessions to minimize possible problems. You may want to schedule shorter sessions, if that's all that your child can handle. If your child can't stand to lose, set up activities rather than competitive games. If your child has trouble taking turns, pick something the kids can all do at the same time.

If your child is more interested in objects than people, and can't wait to play with another child's toys, plan carefully with the other parents involved. You may want to prepare your child, Mary, by explaining that playmate Sally is going to bring over her new doll. Mary can have a turn with the doll, while Sally has a turn with one of Mary's dolls. Make it clear to Mary that she'll need to give Sally's doll back after her turn. Sally's parent can share the same information with Sally. If both girls know what to expect, you're programming the session for success.

You may even want to write a short "social story" about the play session that describes the event the way you want it to go. Each of the girls is a character in the story. You can even put yourself and the other parent it in, praising the girls for playing so well together.

Finally, apply praise with a bucket, not a brush. When we were priming our son Drew to act in a certain ways in various situations in his younger years, we'd praise him lavishly when he did what he was supposed to do. If we accidently neglected this reward on occasion, he wasn't shy about prompting us with some version of, "I did it right, didn't I?" We were quick to agree.

As your child progresses, you can introduce more complex situations to build on his success. Keep in mind that you're helping him learn the lessons he needs to get along in the world at a pace he can handle.

It may take a lot of hours and effort on your part to help your child develop skills that come to other kids intuitively. But consider that your determination, patience and commitment are teaching your child a lesson that can help him build not just social skills, but also a critical armor of self esteem.

Recently, I spoke with a mother who has a daughter with Asperger Syndrome. She said her daughter had always believed in herself, but her experiences in middle school were wearing at that confidence.

The time and effort we invest in our kids, especially if invested continually with enthusiasm and patience, shows them we believe in them. That helps them believe in themselves, because they're getting the message through actions as well as words.

And every one of those actions is a step toward making that big picture we hold in our heads -- the one of a positive, successful life for our children -- a reality.

###

39 ASPERGER SYNDROME: PUT THOSE KIDS TO WORK!

We'd do anything for our kids with Asperger Syndrome.

Is that always a good thing? Hmmmmmm. Hard to say. It's good if we can figure out what we need to do for our kids versus what they need to do for themselves. And that's not always easy. Maybe an outside view would be good. I talked with the director of a high school job placement program for special needs kids and she laid it on the line, "I think these kids are too often...well...babied. They need to do more for themselves."

You should know that this program director, Mary Beth Berry, cares passionately about her charges. She's amazingly persuasive at getting employers to give the kids in her program real work experience during part of their school day. She's an expert at job coaching and building confidence. I respect her opinion.

How many of us sometimes think of our kids as chicks with broken wings? How many sometimes have horrible visions of plummeting crashes if we push them out of the nest to do things on their own?

Let's think back on our lives. Didn't we learn some of our most important lessons from our failures? Are our kids really that fragile? Sure, there are thoughtless people in the world, but there are also great, helpful folks out there. And we're not going to be around forever. And our kids can't succeed until they try.

Another job expert I spoke with, Asperger Syndrome advocate Dr. Peter Gerhardt, talked about helping a young man learn to ride the train to work. They talked about it. They rode the train together. But finally the day came when the young man had to ride to work alone. Peter said that if he could have run next to the train all the way to the job, he would have. But it went fine. And that daily commute became a normal part of the young man's work life.

As Peter says, work is a defining characteristic of our lives. One of the first questions we're asked when we meet someone is, "What do you do?"

What they mean, of course is, "What's your job?" If people with Asperger Syndrome don't have the opportunity to work, they're cut off from a key part of life, not to mention a way to support themselves.

Okay, we're all sold on the importance of work. Now here's part two. And it's a biggie. We want our sons and daughters to work. They want to work. But how do they find and hold a job? Unemployment is distressingly high among people with AS. How do you beat the odds?

You start early.

Take the attitude that your child, at whatever skill level, is going to work. Talk about jobs and get him thinking about what he'd like to do. Does your son want to do something that sounds impossible? Be realistic, but aim high. He may not become an astronaut, but maybe he could work at NASA, or maybe at an airport. Of course, some people may be extremely happy filing reports for a living, and that's great, especially if organizing is your child's passion.

Our kids tend to have intense special interests and often have extraordinary abilities. If we can channel these qualities into a paying career, we've hit the motherlode. So wherever you go, encourage your daughter to look at people working and consider if she'd like those jobs. Encourage her to talk with people about their jobs. What are the job's responsibilities and duties? What education or training do you need? What are the good and bad things about the job?

Help your kids understand the job interview process and what an employer is looking for. Get a book or magazine about applying for a job and help your children learn the process.

Help them learn to realistically understand their strengths and challenges and how to advocate for themselves.

Most of all, get them some work experience as soon as possible. Paid or unpaid. During school vacations, if just managing schoolwork is all-consuming. The best way to learn work skills is to work, whether your child is going directly from high school to a job, or plans on going to college or vocational training first. Remember, there's a lot more to working than specific job duties. A large part of a job can be arriving on time, following directions, staying on task, knowing safety procedures, getting along with co-workers and other "surround" issues.

Let's revisit the chick-from-the-nest analogy. The best crash avoidance we can offer is flight training. We can make sure that our kids' Individual Education Plans include transition planning beginning at age 14 as required by the Individuals with Disabilities Education Act. We can work with our kids' schools and with social service agencies to help our kids find part-time jobs during their high school years with understanding employers. Job coaches can help our kids learn a job until they're ready to go solo.

And we can train our kids to increasingly advocate for themselves so that when they look for a job on their own, they can present themselves as the kind of capable, hardworking employees businesses want to hire. And, if necessary, they can educate their employers about how AS affects them and negotiate any needed accommodations.

We won't go into detail here discussing the Americans with Disabilities Act, reasonable accommodations and disclosure issues. Think of that as homework.

Today, let's just get determined to get our sons and daughters real work experience as early as possible.

When my son was diagnosed with Asperger Syndrome, my wife and I had a lot of questions, including: could he ever hold a job? Now, he's a veteran of two successful part-time jobs and is working toward a career in forensic science.

He's already accomplished more than we -– in our worst moments -– ever thought possible. Here's a lesson: don't let your worst fears limit your kids.

Let's give them some preparation, give them some safety nets, but get them out there — and give them the chance to blast past our expectations.

###

40 WRITING KIDS OFF IS NOT AN OPTION

If you're a parent or teacher or coach or youth leader, have you ever been tempted to write a child off? To expect little or nothing and put your efforts elsewhere? For an hour or a day or even permanently? Have you ever felt justified because a child was uncooperative or disinterested or disruptive?

This can be a particular temptation when you have other children or students who need you and show more appreciation for your efforts and make more progress. But it's also an opportunity to be one of those special people who never gives up on a child. Who never mentally throws up his hands and says, "It's his own fault, he's not even trying."

In John Elder Robison's book, "Look Me In The Eye: My Life With Asperger's," he writes about being frequently written off as a child. He makes the point that his parents and teachers and psychologists often misunderstood his intentions. For example, he said that child psychologists who said "John prefers to play by himself," got it dead wrong.

"I never wanted to be alone...I played by myself because I was a failure at playing with others. I was alone as a result of my own limitations, and being alone was one of the bitterest disappointments of my young life."

Although he became highly successful in later life as he learned to interact with people on their terms, Robison says he will always carry the pain of people routinely misunderstanding and criticizing and rejecting him when he was young.

Many children with Asperger Syndrome, autism or other neurobiological conditions have behaviors that are easy to misinterpret. Many try hard to succeed, but their brains process information differently than most other kids.

Some may blurt out answers in class. Some get frustrated and have meltdowns at things that are trivial to other children.

It's not enough to tell these kids the rules, because their brains are operating from a separate set of rules that seem right to them. A child who disrupts a class (from your point of view) may be desperately trying to participate. A child who tells other children what to do, may absolutely believe he is helping them. Even a child who sometimes needs to be alone, because too much sensory stimulation can be overwhelming, may also yearn to interact with other kids. Sometimes it takes a die-hard parent or teacher or leader to help these kids learn and relate so they can succeed in life.

I'm not talking about throwing out discipline and consequences. I'm talking about applying the rules with compassion and making accommodations while you help a child see things from a perspective that's foreign to him. About trying to find out what a child is thinking and why she acts the way she does. About seeking help if dealing with a special needs child, along with other children, becomes overwhelming.

Writing a child off is getting stuck on what we can't do with him or her. What if we always focus, instead, on what else we could try? What if we live by the approach adopted by the mission control crew in the movie "Apollo 13," when three astronauts' lives were at stake?

"Failure is not an option."

###

41 ONE SIZE FITS ONE

Your child is unique. Yes, that's true for every parent. But parents of children with Asperger Syndrome or autism may feel it's an understatement. Unique means one of a kind. But our kids are often…turbo unique. One of a kind with extra difference sauce.

And the world can be very unforgiving of differences. Or rather, with no malice intended, the world is often just not set up to deal with the different.

I've run into challenges just being tall. At the first college I attended, it was mandatory for men to enroll in ROTC, the U.S. Army's Reserve Officer Training Corps. We were issued uniforms to wear during early morning marching drills.

As I stood in line to get my uniform, with my 6 foot 4 inch height and size 14 feet, I discovered first hand that the Army was not into accommodations. When they didn't have a uniform long enough, they just handed me the closest they had, inches too short in the sleeves and the pant-legs. But the shoes were the real triumph of anti-accommodation. Not having a size 14, they gave me the biggest they had, an extra-wide pair of size 12s.

Was I supposed to fold my feet in sideways to make them fit? To be fair, the army was not actively trying to torture me. The uniforms were bought to fit people within a common range of sizes and there was no system in place to deal with exceptions. It was my problem, not theirs.

I sometimes see schools expecting our kids to conform to one-size-fits-all classroom rules and routines in the way I was expected to cram my feet into my army-issued footwear. As I recall, I tried, and limped through one long drill session. After that, I wore black loafers and took the demerits for showing up in non-regulation shoes.

The other day, I heard about a mother who'd asked her child's teacher if she could acquire an extra set of school books for her son because he had trouble bringing them home. The teacher refused, saying if she allowed one child to have them, everyone in the class would want them. After presenting a doctor's note, the mom prevailed.

Of course, we don't expect schools to accept dangerous or highly disruptive behaviors or focus attention on our children to the exclusion of others. Unfortunately, there are many completely reasonable accommodations (many included in Individual Education Plans) that some teachers resist because they don't understand that a child truly needs them. Also, a significant number of schools are based on a mass-production factory model. Find what works best for the most children and use it. My son attended such a school in a suburb of Atlanta.

Luckily, even in factory-like school systems, I've heard parents tell of teachers who are open minded, flexible and willing to adapt the rules to find the best way to help each individual student. As parents, we love these teachers. We praise them to the skies. We want to clone them.

Well, why not?

If we can't exactly clone them, we can influence their school systems to set them up as role models.

If your child has a superb teacher, make sure your school's administration knows what a great job she or he is doing. Write positive letters to your school's principal. Then write to your school system's superintendent or school board. Write an open letter to your local newspaper. Be specific about what this teacher has done and how your child has benefited. Seek out other parents who are also pleased and encourage them to write similar letters.

I've worked extensively in both corporations and schools. Complaint letters are frequently dealt with at lower levels, but everybody likes to show letters of praise to an organization's leaders.

This can encourage your school system to hold your treasured teacher up as an example to other teachers, or even to include that teacher's attributes in future performance expectations for the entire staff. Even if you can't clone a great teacher's natural abilities, the next best thing is to influence other teachers to use his or her methods.

This is just one step toward making our schools more accepting of differences, but it can be an effective one.

There's no way we can always protect our children from situations where they have to take the demerits for being different. But the more teachers we have actively supporting reasonable accommodations and flexibility, the more classrooms we can make into "demerit free difference zones."

And that's a one-size-fits-one kind of environment that can free a child's spirit.

###

42 KNOWING WHAT WE DON'T KNOW

Miscommunication.

We're all guilty of it. Believing what we've said is perfectly clear and then learning that a family member misunderstood. This is a special hazard when someone in the family has Asperger Syndrome and a brain that processes information in a highly individual way.

Here's an example.

When my son, Drew, went away to college, his mom and I offered him a lot of advice. Among other things, we suggested he use his college's academic support center. This was a service that helped students review their assignments, understand what was required, and then coach them to do their best work. Drew had always done well in school, but because he has Asperger Syndrome, his mom and I figured, "He's living away from home for the first time, so he can use all the academic support he can get."

Drew reluctantly agreed.

He settled into college life and we were pleased that he was succeeding, not just academically, but socially. We'd occasionally think of and ask about the academic support center, but Drew never seemed to get around to going. His overall grades were good enough that it wasn't a priority, so we didn't press the issue.

In his junior year, when we were helping him make decisions about changing his major, we learned the reason for his reluctance. We'd assumed that Drew had the same understanding of the academic support center that we did. But he'd thought it was a counseling center and that counselors there would ask him questions and report back to his mom. Sort of remote-control parental supervision. Drew was reveling in his independence. The last thing he wanted was more supervision.

For Drew, living away from home, managing his own life and graduating from college was a major accomplishment. While he did great in some classes and spent four years in his school's honors program, there were other courses he struggled with early on. The academic support center could have helped him.

While this was not a sink or swim situation, it was a lesson to me to assume less and discuss more in family interactions. More than once over the years (and by "more than once," I mean, frequently) my wife has warned me about my tendency to lecture to our kids. What I saw as friendly, helpful counsel learned from experience, she saw as advising them until their eyes glazed over. At least she stopped short of using the word, "rant."

Anyway, the academic support center episode helped me understand that, when I talk, I need to continually think about asking for feedback to make sure my family members understand what I mean. And that I may need to ask extra questions to make sure I understand what they mean. They make assumptions, too.

It's not enough to know. We also have to make the effort to know what we don't know. You know?

###

43 REWRITING YOUR CHILD'S SCRIPT

There's a term in screenwriting called "the dark night of the soul." It's that point in the script where the hero is overwhelmed by feelings that he faces impossible odds and his situation is hopeless.

If your child with Asperger Syndrome is frequently seized by these feelings, they may be caused by thoughts of past embarrassing or traumatic incidents that are taking up too much space in his memory banks.

Some children with AS, including my son, Drew, are especially sensitive to selective memories. Here's an example. When Drew was about three and a half years old, he got a balloon tied to his wrist in a shoe store. While walking to the car, he accidently untied the balloon's string and it floated away, followed by his desperate cries. This event had such an impact on him that for years afterward, he would get extremely upset if anyone offered to give him a balloon. Drew explained recently that the balloon was a beautiful thing, he had to watch it fly away while there was nothing he could do -- and he never wanted to feel that way again.

This was only a lost balloon. For a child with Asperger Syndrome who's remembering being teased or harassed, or failing at something important to him, the rush of emotions can be overwhelming. They can play over and over in a loop that tells a child that it's impossible to succeed or be happy.

Even a child who has an overall positive outlook and lots of abilities can be subject to these bouts of negativity and depression.

It's impossible to know what's going to trigger bad memories and start such a loop, but you can help your child break it. You do it by showing him how to rewrite the script in his head.

And it takes a rewrite. You can't just erase the memory like you'd delete lines in a script.

Telling a child not to think about a bad memory is like someone saying to you, "Don't think about elephants." No matter how hard you try, a picture of a pachyderm will pop into your head.

Instead, work with your child to prepare a list of positive memories to hold ready. That way, when a negative memory surfaces, he can direct his thoughts to the time he made a great presentation in class, or solved a difficult puzzle, or accomplished something else that made him proud.

It's best if the positive memories focus on accomplishments, because they're evidence of competence and self-worth that can be powerful at refuting negative thoughts.

If you can't help your child learn to redirect negative thoughts and you see that he frequently gets down on himself, you may want to consider getting professional help.

But working yourself to build up your son or daughter is never a wasted effort.

Sitting with your child to compile a list of his accomplishments and good memories is a treat in and of itself. And you're teaching your child that it's always possible to take control of his own script, and write the positive story he deserves.

###

Dan Coulter

SUCCEEDING AT PARENTING

44 BECOMING BULLETPROOF PARENTS

Ever been frustrated or embarrassed by something one of your kids said or did in public? The stares of strangers can feel like bullets. If your child has an Autism Spectrum Disorder, you may sometimes feel like you've been machine-gunned.

Wouldn't it be great to have a way to deal with these situations that made you bulletproof?

I found something that works sort of like a protective shield — and it's basically a matter of perspective.

Most of us were raised to care a lot about what other people think. That's generally a good thing. It helps us be aware of social rules and interact politely with other people. But when our kids do something embarrassing in public, feeling those painful stares can sometimes cause us to get our priorities mixed up.

Maybe your son throws tantrums. Maybe your daughter makes inappropriate remarks in a loud voice. When my son, who has Asperger Syndrome, was little, he had a tendency to pick up and examine anything that caught his interest. This was a problem, particularly in stores.

People react in a lot of ways to their kids "misbehaving" in public. Too often, I've seen parents act embarrassed and say things to their kids that they might regret later. Most of us don't completely lose it, but I know there were times when my son was little that I was more impatient with him in public than I should have been.

Now for the perspective part. At the moment our kids do something in public that we wish they hadn't, we're socially conditioned to react by focusing on what other people think. But how important is that compared to what our kids need at that moment? Do you have a picture of anyone in the mall crowd on your dresser at home? Have you held anyone in the supermarket line in your arms and rocked him to sleep? Is anyone in sight more important to you than your child?

When you look at things from that perspective, it's easier to dismiss what other people think and focus on your child. First off, why did he do what he did? Many kids with ASDs are impulsive. Something in their brain triggers a behavior that's hard for them to control. What if your son is not defying you? What if he's responding to a stimulus that may take a lot of practice to overcome? In my son's case, it helped to remind him before we went out that he needed to ask and get permission before he picked things up to check them out. We'd remind him again just before we went into a store. Even so, it took quite a while for him to gain control of that behavior.

Knowing that our kids are prone to certain behaviors helps us mentally prepare to stop what we're doing and deal calmly with the situation. There's a saying in the retail business, "Customers are not an interruption of our work, they are the reason for it." I think the same thing applies to parents and kids. Our job of parenting doesn't stop when we're busy and stressed and in a supermarket -- and kids aren't reduced to "interruptions." If your daughter grabs a piece of candy from a shelf and screams when you try and take it from her, the best thing for her may be for you to stop shopping for a moment, kneel down and patiently but firmly explain why she has to put it back. At that moment, being bulletproof to what others might think of her outburst protects you both.

We don't flip a switch to teach our kids and then flip if off. We're teaching them with every interaction we have. If I think of every exchange with my son as one he may remember the rest of his life, will I act differently?

The twist to this is that stopping to deal compassionately and fairly with your child will probably make people who witness his behavior appreciate your parenting skills. And if they don't understand, that's their loss.

Do we care what other people think? Sure. But never as much as we care about our kids.

45 CHEERLEADING FOR PARENTS

I've had a taste of acclaim a number of times in my life.

The first time that stands out was riding on the bus to an "away" basketball game in junior high school. The cheerleaders were doing that "Bill, Bill, he's our man, if he can't do it, David can…" thing where they go through the names of everyone on the team. Even though I was on the second string and the girl leading the cheer had to refer to the program at each name to make sure she didn't miss anyone, it was very heady stuff to hear, "Stan, Stan, he's our man, if he can't do it, Dan can! Dan, Dan, He's our man…" Of course, it was only five seconds of fame, followed by the unsettling assurance that if I couldn't do it, the next guy down the roster could. Still, for those few seconds, I got to hear my name chanted by a busload of cheerleaders and imagine I was the subject of hero worship.

Everyone could use that kind of positive reinforcement once in a while. Trouble is, we rarely get it when we most deserve it.

This week, I was reading an autism-related magazine and was really drawn into an article about parents who were devoting tremendous amounts of time and effort to helping their kids who are on the spectrum. I admired these parents. They really deserved to be written up, especially in a magazine that's read by people who can appreciate their situation.

It made me think about all the other parents of kids on the spectrum who are trying their best, but often get met with criticism or misunderstanding.

Raising a child who's on the autism spectrum is tough. To be fair, it's hard for anyone who hasn't been involved to understand just how tough it is. When my son, Drew, was in grade school, he hadn't yet been diagnosed with Asperger Syndrome. We were working under the diagnoses of "communication handicapped" and "ADHD." I remember talking with a colleague at my office, describing his difficult behaviors. Her reaction was, "But isn't that just normal boy stuff?" No echoes of cheerleaders chanting my name in that conversation.

Because most people don't understand what's involved, we parents of kids on the spectrum have a smaller universe of people who can appreciate what we do. I was talking with Lori Shery, president of the ASPEN support group, the other day about the things that special needs support groups have to offer. One of the things she mentioned was sharing our kids' accomplishments at meetings, "Other parents might say, 'Well, that's no big deal,' but it is, it's a very big deal to us."

People who don't appreciate what's involved can't give us the positive reinforcement that can help us through the tough times. The more alone you are, the easier it is to doubt yourself or wonder if you're making the right decisions.

That's why I think it's important to be a part of a community of people who understand. While we're working to educate the world about our kids, it really helps to be in contact with people who already have a clue.

Support groups can be great. We're members of the ASPEN organization, the MAAP organization and the local chapter of the Autism Society of America, among others. ASPEN and MAAP focus on higher-functioning conditions on the autism spectrum, such as Asperger Syndrome, while the ASA addresses the entire spectrum.

Because we've been involved with ASPEN the longest, I'll say a few words about how it's helped us. We joined a local ASPEN chapter while we lived in New Jersey and kept our membership when we moved to North Carolina. In New Jersey, my wife, Julie, and I took turns going to the meetings so one of us could stay home with our kids. I remember how reassuring the ASPEN meetings were; especially right after Drew was diagnosed. Professionals came to the meetings to speak and answer questions. Later, parents could trade info and compare notes. Every time we realized we were doing something right, it helped lower our anxiety level.

I also subscribe to a number of online autism-related forums where people share information, concerns and support. Online forums are great because you can access them from wherever you live.

So here's my pitch.

Let's all make it a point to compliment another parent every chance we get on what he or she is doing. I don't mean just when you see them do something outstanding. Look for something they're doing that you agree with or admire and let them know. Maybe you'll tell a support group leader you really appreciate her volunteering to organize and run meetings. Maybe you'll tell another parent who shared a difficulty that you appreciate how he dealt with the situation. Maybe you'll hug your spouse and say how much you appreciate his or her patience. But look for opportunities to give that jolt of encouragement and approval.

It costs us nothing, but it can mean the world. And praising others may just spark someone to tell you what a great job you're doing when you really need to hear it.

If the moment's really special, you may just capture that junior high school feeling of having a whole squad of cheerleaders chanting your name.

I bet you deserve it.

###

46 REDUCING SPECIAL NEEDS PARENT STRESS

A lot of parents who have kids with special needs get a free helping of stress every day. With extra nuts -- and sprinkles.

If this is you, how do you start an anti-stress diet? Start small. Take a break.

Oh yeah, right. When are you going to find the time?

Most of us have heard we'd be more efficient if we'd take a break once in a while. But it's hard to convince your brain that taking some time to ease your stress will really help you get more done. Mr. Brain often stubbornly sees things in the short term. If you've got 1000 orders to process and it takes about a minute to process an order, taking a five-minute break every hour means you process fewer orders in an eight hour day and fall farther behind, right?

Nope.

I read a study a while back that showed when data-processing workers got a five-minute break every hour, they had less stress and got more work done in an eight-hour day. The benefits of the break more than made up for the time away from the computer.

Here's the really interesting part of the story: in spite of the findings, the company associated with the study did NOT start giving their data processing workers five-minute breaks each hour. Huh? The bosses couldn't bring themselves to do it. In spite of the evidence, it just seemed counterproductive.

Maybe your brain is working from the same perspective, with a side of guilt thrown in. Have you ever kept at a task way past the point of diminishing returns because you were working on behalf of your family and it seemed like you'd be short-changing them to take even a few minutes for yourself?

Part of the problem is that when you're overloaded and stress is building, that stress can affect your judgment. Stress can put you in a hole and make it hard to see a way to climb out. So you work and work and get more tired and frustrated and make mistakes – and sometimes get sick.

As I write this, I'm looking at a National Institute for Occupational Safety and Health (NIOSH) study http://www.cdc.gov/niosh/docs/99-101/ that says health care expenditures are nearly 50% greater for workers who report high levels of stress.

So there's a reason to relax you can relate to! You can't do as good a job taking care of your kids if you're sick – so consider being your own doctor and ordering yourself to relax a bit.

By the way, here are a few of the conditions that the NIOSH study says contribute to stress:

"...heavy workload, infrequent rest breaks, long work hours...conflicting or uncertain job expectations, too much responsibility, too many "hats to wear"...lack of support or help... rapid changes for which workers are unprepared..."

Doesn't that sort of sound like a job description for a parent of a special needs child?

If you're feeling stretched too thin, here are some suggestions to improve your life and get more done by taking some time for yourself: (NOTE: If you feel like you can't manage your stress by yourself, I'd suggest you seek professional help. Try these recommendations if you're confident you can take some positive steps on your own.)

RELAXATION TIPS

When you're starting a task, set an alarm or kitchen timer to go off in an hour. When it goes off, take a five-minute break. Stand up, stretch, walk outside. Do something that gets your mind off the task for a few minutes. Each time you start to work again, reset that timer so you get a few minutes every hour to recharge your batteries. (My wife gave me a desk clock that chimes on the hour to remind me to take breaks.)

If you're working long days, it's also good to take a 15 minute break every few hours.

Don't neglect lunch. Taking a half-hour or an hour off for lunch can be a real energizer in the middle of a busy day. If possible, do some socializing during lunch, either in person or on the phone.

Find some favorite songs and listen to them during your breaks. A song you like can really help get your mind off work for a few minutes. Another option is to stand up and stretch, then sit in your chair, close your eyes and take five slow, deep breaths.

If at all possible, take a daily walk. A 20 to 30 minute daily walk can help reduce your stress and help you get or stay fit. I'm a lot calmer since I started walking. Ask my wife. I look forward to it so much that I make it a priority and find ways to work it into a busy day.

When you feel yourself getting stressed to the point where you keep spinning your wheels, try shifting your brain into neutral for a while. Let things wash over you. Some decisions won't wait, but if you're upset and you can postpone a decision, it's usually a good idea to calm down first. This may save you from saying something you regret or doing something you wish you could undo. When you're spinning your wheels in frustration, a little neutral time can help you find a way to get traction that you hadn't noticed because your stress gave you a blind spot.

Get out a calendar and plan some time for yourself. Going out one night a week for a few hours can help put some balance and perspective into your life. Don't you feel and work better when you have something to look forward to? If you and your spouse can do it together, great. If not, take turns. If you're a single parent, maybe you can trade off with another single parent.

Go out with friends or see a movie by yourself — whatever you enjoy. If you can't make it every week, make it every other week. One thing is sure: you have to take the initiative and give yourself permission. Don't be apologetic. You're not goofing off. You're making an investment in a person who is crucial to your family: you.

In my experience, these pauses for relaxation can help make you more efficient, more optimistic and give you ideas you just can't get when the fatigue poisons are building up in your brain.

It may seem hard to find the time at first, but a little relaxation can make you a better mom or dad.

So you really have no choice.

Your kids deserve it.

###

47 LISTENING TO YOUR KIDS

How are you listening to your kids?

If you're one of those rare "born listeners" who can get almost anyone to open up, you're lucky. If you're like the rest of us, you can probably improve your listening skills.

Maybe you're frustrated that your kids don't give you a chance to listen. Do you get a one-word response when you ask how the day went at school? "Fine." And don't your instincts often tell you that "fine" is a wildly inaccurate description of the day?

You might be making one of the mistakes I made for years. I used to interrupt. A lot. And I didn't realize what I was doing. It's also easy to lecture - and to have an answer for everything.

But look at this from your son or daughter's perspective. Sometimes it's hard to describe a situation in words. Things are often more complicated than you can convey in a couple of sentences. If a person you talk to routinely interrupts you or criticizes you or tells you what to do, you may feel he's making pronouncements on a situation he doesn't fully understand.

And that can train you not to confide in that person. So, you might be unintentionally training your child not to share things with you.

Attentive listening generates respect. Several years ago, I interviewed a number of successful public relations people for a documentary on PR counseling. Hal Burson -- founding chairman of Burson-Marsteller, the world's largest PR firm -- told an interesting story, "I have had any number of experiences throughout my own work where I would go visit a CEO, spend 30, 40 minutes, an hour with that CEO, and he would do all of the talking. And I would ask a question every now and then, and then two days later the reports would get back to me, 'that guy Burson's a really smart guy'."

Maybe we should counsel our kids more like CEOs and pay attention in a way that gains their "listening respect" before we offer advice or direction.

Think of it as taking the long road and not the short cut. In the short cut, we listen just enough to get a picture of the situation and then jump in to make our comments and provide our brilliant guidance.

When we take the long road, we may ask questions to draw out the speaker or guide the conversation, but we hold off on conclusions. Even when we feel a burning desire, we bite back interjections such as, "What did you do that for?" or "You should have." or "Next time you need to."

This can be hard. We're the adults. But maybe that's part of the problem. As long as we treat our kids like - well, kids - it's tempting to just tell them what to do. We've got the experience! If they'd just listen to us!

But even good advice can roll off kids like a quick shower runs off a lawn. When we really listen and ask questions that can help our kids come up with solutions on their own, it's more like a long shower that soaks in and reaches the roots.

When I was growing up, some friends of mine had parents who were good listeners. They'd hear me out without assuming they knew the end of the story. It felt like they were listening to me as they'd listen to another adult. It made me want to act more like an adult in my conversation - and really think things through.

There's tremendous power in listening. Sometimes we just need to talk something through to understand it better ourselves. What a gift it is to find someone who doesn't automatically start offering solutions as though our problems have easy answers that we just aren't smart enough to think of ourselves.

And after we've been fully attentive, we'll probably find our children are more willing to listen to the subtle guidance we're bursting to offer. We could even (GASP) ask if they would like to hear our thoughts. Of course, for serious issues where we feel it's required, we can always lay down the law. And maybe even that will work better when our kids think they've had a fair hearing and that we understand what we're talking about.

The sooner we start - and the younger our kids - the better. It can be hard to regain the "listening trust" of a teenager who's learned to be very careful responding to parental inquiries. (Mom's asking a question! SHIELDS UP!) But it can be done.

That's my 2 cents worth.

Hey, thanks for listening. And for not interrupting. You know, after this little talk, I realize - you're a really smart parent.

###

48 TEACHING WHAT MATTERS

Wouldn't the world be a better place if our kids hung on our every word? If they worshiped our wisdom and lived to do everything we told them to do?

Probably not, but it's easy to feel that way. And it's so tempting to try and impart our gems of wisdom as they come to us. Often we do exactly that, as if we were applying post-it notes to our kids' bodies, expecting them to keep each note handy and reach out and find exactly the right advice at the right time.

Like that's going to happen.

So do we always have the right to get frustrated when they do something we've told them not to do - or fail to do something we now expect of them? For many kids, I think getting ad hoc advice as it pops into their parents' heads must be more like getting peppered with pebbles. The pebbles are annoying and most of them just bounce off.

This all came to mind as my wife and I talked with our son, who has Asperger Syndrome, on the last day of his winter college break. We were bursting with advice and ideas on things Drew could do to improve his study habits, keep his room cleaner, store his clean laundry differently...and on and on.

We had our advice pebble slingshots out and had started peppering our son before we came to our senses and got realistic. We wound up talking about just a few things we'd like him to do differently and discussed practical ways he could make these changes.

This was much more in line with the way his brain absorbs information. Like many kids, he has a hard time changing habits he's developed over a long time. A habit is like a template in your head. If you want to change the behavior, you have to rewrite the template - and that takes time and effort.

So it makes sense to pick the most important habits you want your child to learn -- or to unlearn -- and work on them one at a time. One of the things we focused on while Drew was home this college break was using email. He routinely uses instant messaging to talk with his friends, but has had a hard time remembering to check his email on a regular basis. This was not only frustrating to us as parents, but had the potential to cause problems at school. His college instructors and administrators often communicate with students through email. So not checking email meant risking not knowing about assignment changes or school announcements.

Our solution was to send him emails while he was home and remind him to check them every day to help him get in the habit. Also, when I drove him back to school, we set up his computer to automatically open his email program every time he turned on his computer as a reminder to check for messages.

My wife and I were delighted when he began promptly responding to our emails -- and ecstatic when he began generating his own. We heaped on the praise in subsequent email messages.

That's important too. Sometimes it's easy to use on our kids what we used to call "exception reporting" when I worked for the phone company. "Exception reporting," means only getting a report when something goes wrong. If your kids only hear from you when you're telling them what they need to change, you're probably not a lot of fun to be around. You may also get tuned out a lot.

We've found some of the most important things to work on with Drew involved safety skills and self-advocacy skills. Safety skills include more than avoiding physical danger. We've talked with him about scams and not giving out personal or financial info on the Internet. We've also talked about how he needs to approach his instructors to make sure he understands assignments and knows what he needs to focus on to do the best possible job in a course.

Yes, we'd like his room to be neater and cleaner, but as long as he's not breeding deadly E. coli or typhoid, we're not likely to start staging surprise inspections.

The clichés "pick your battles" and "don't sweat the small stuff" have their roots in sound reasoning. Think about the skills that are most important for your son or daughter to learn to live independently. These are probably the most important things you can work on. And it's much easier - as we've learned - to work on these things while your kids are still living at home.

Test runs are also invaluable. Telling your child how to do something pales in comparison with showing him and then having him do it himself. Many of our kids also need to have complex actions broken down into clear steps.

For example, making a purchase in a store's checkout line involves:
1. Selecting your item or items.
2. Checking their prices and making sure you have enough money to buy them.
3. Finding the checkout counter and standing in line.
4. Keeping focused in line. Remembering who you're standing behind and moving forward when that person moves.

5. When you reach the checkout clerk, handing your items to the clerk or putting them on the counter where he or she can reach them.
6. Waiting for the clerk to total your purchases and tell you how much you owe.
7. Handing the clerk enough money to pay for the purchases.
8. Waiting for the clerk to hand you your change, if you have any coming.
9. Waiting for the clerk to put your purchase in a bag, if it requires a bag or if the store's checkout clerks just routinely bag merchandise.
10. Taking your purchase and your receipt with you when you leave the checkout counter and the store.

When Drew was young and learning about shopping, he was easily distracted and didn't always remember to step forward as a checkout line moved up. I also observed him handing his money to the clerk with his merchandise instead of waiting for the clerk to ring up his purchase. With some guidance and practice, he absorbed his "checkout etiquette" and was able to go shopping on his own with no problem. Letting him handle checkout chores whenever it was practical during shopping trips helped build his skills and confidence. There's no substitute for letting your child do all these steps himself, only stepping in to assist if you absolutely have to, and giving him or her immediate feedback afterwards.

It's never too early to identify key life skills and start practicing the most important ones. Working consistently on these "core skills" will be much more effective than just peppering your kids with advice as it pops into your head.

As for all those unused pebbles of wisdom, I'm thinking of using mine to build a life-size replica of the Great Wall of China. Now if I can just figure out what to do with all the leftovers...

###

49 THE POWER OF FUN

We tend to remember extremes: our best days and worst days.

You usually can't control the worst days. Bad stuff happens when it happens.

But you can make more days some of your family's best days by recognizing and harnessing the power of fun. It can bring your family closer, help you teach your kids what you want them to learn and get you all through tough times.

Just about everyone knows someone who's fun to be around. Maybe it's an aunt or uncle or someone you've worked with. Someone who seems to generate laughter and good times.

Picture yourself playing that role for your family.

Maybe you're already a walking fun factory. If not, and this just doesn't sound like you, hear me out. I'm not talking about a personality transplant or suggesting that you assume a forced goofiness. I'm talking about focusing on the part of us all that enjoys having fun. Wherever you are on the fun scale, you can probably turn it up a notch.

I have, at different times in my life, been Mr. Fun and a real downer to be around. Finding ways to snap myself out of a bad mood became a crucial skill when my kids came into my life. Especially when I was working long hours and only saw them at the end of the day and on weekends. I couldn't afford to waste any time with them moping around.

Every family is different, but let me share a few things we've done to generate fun.

When my kids were little, I never did learn to completely leave work pressures at the office, but I'd juice myself up on the way home thinking about being with them and my wife, Julie.

When I hit the door, I'd pick up both Drew and Jessie and dance around the hallway, singing a little rapid-fire nonsense song I'd made up. They got a tremendous kick out of it, and it set a great tone for the rest of the evening. I found out early that things are only as special as you make them.

When things are tough or strained, a little fun can help turn things around. I remember working in my home-office on a weekend and hearing Julie, calling up the stairs, asking me if I could take some time and help her. She was dealing with housework and our two toddler kids and she was more than a bit exasperated. I grabbed a portable tape recorder and shoved in a tape of the William Tell Overture, also used as the theme from "The Lone Ranger" on television. Many of you may recognize this as standard "rescue" music on old film soundtracks. Anyway, I rushed down the stairs like a comic book superhero with the William Tell Overture playing at full blast. I don't remember what I was working on at the time, but I know putting it aside and making a big entrance to immediately pitch in on family matters was a huge hit with Julie and the kids.

Playing family games was fun for us. I think one of the keys to success is monkeying with the rules so everyone can play. You don't have to throw the rules out the window, just modify them so young kids or those with some challenges can fully participate.

It's a hoot to play Scrabble with made-up words allowed - as long as they're inventive and you make up a fun meaning.

Pictionary, a kind of drawing version of "charades," was our favorite for a while. My kids still kid me about a duck I drew that looked like anything but.

One of Julie's real strengths is coming up with great gifts. She puts real thought into family presents. She also loves to bake and present the kids with care packages of brownies, cookies, cheese straws and such. No mama ever showered her kids with more encouragement than my wife - and I can always count on hearing her laughing when she's on the phone with Drew or Jessie.

We also had a lot of fun with bedtime stories. My son and daughter were born 17 months apart, so they were close enough in age to enjoy many of the same things at the same time, such as bedtime stories.

Every night when they were old enough to enjoy them, I'd make up a new story for Drew and Jessie. Until I decided to tape record the stories so I could offer the kids "reruns" when I felt too tired to come up with new ideas.

Not that the stories were all original. I borrowed liberally from any book, movie play, TV show or cartoon I'd ever seen for ideas. The tape recordings are testaments to how tired I was many nights, because you can hear me yawn frequently during the stories. But those recordings are a treasure now. Not so much for what I'm saying, but for the laughs and questions and suggestions from my kids that are sprinkled throughout the soundtrack. There's a story on one tape which features Drew as a prince and Jessie as a princess. In passing, my voice notes that Princess Jessie has on a beautiful dress. I move quickly on toward a peak of adventure when Jessie interrupts and hauls me back. "What about the dwess?" her little voice chirps. She had her own priorities. Adventure could, and did, wait for a detailed description of the princess dress.

The stories featured Jessie's stuffed teddy bear, "Bearly." Bearly Bear would routinely pop into Jessie's room and lead Jessie and Drew through a magic door in Jessie's closet to the land of the Bear King. The Bear King's realm was frequently invaded by evil wizards, who'd have to be out-smarted and banished by Jessie, Drew and Bearly. Professional note: Evil wizards are particularly vulnerable to having dirty socks thrust beneath their noses. It makes them swoon so you can knock off their wizard hats and cut them off from their sources of power. You get the idea.

When my wife and I take long car trips, I like to listen to CDs I made of some of these old tapes and hear Drew and Jessie whoop it up in the background when an evil wizard gets a particularly smelly sock shoved in his face at a pivotal point in the story and goes into hysterics.

So, if you have any flair for story telling, I'd milk the dirty sock bit for all it's worth. It's killer material for four and five-year-olds.

And if storytelling's not your forte, no problem. Your local library is chock-full of great children's books you can read to your kids. You can even change the names of characters in the books and substitute your kids' names. Kids love hearing about themselves and librarians can be a huge help in pointing you toward fun books in the right age range. If you have more than one child, it's a great way to help them bond.

When families have a child with a disability, dealing with disability issues for a son or daughter can suck up a lot of time and make your other children feel neglected. Including all your kids in story time can help you wire into their brains that it's fun to be together. Not to mention the opportunity to reinforce any other lessons you want to teach in the stories you tell or read. Having said this, we also found it was important to routinely spend one-on-one time with each of our kids.

Beginning in preschool, Drew was diagnosed with a series of communications-related disorders. He finally got a correct diagnosis of Asperger Syndrome. Even before we knew he had AS, we were trying to address his special needs.

It is a challenge to give both kids "equal time" when one has a special need. But looking back, giving attention to both kids helped bring them and our family closer together. And we had a lot of fun along the way. Fun has made it easier to relate to the kids when they've gotten frustrated, especially when we've needed to persuade them to do something for their health or well-being. Fun is like oil that helps the family gears mesh smoothly.

Fun has been an important factor in our marriage, too. I heard a statistic the other day that the majority of parents who have kids on the autism spectrum get divorced. Finding ways to have fun while you're dealing with overwhelming pressure is like a life preserver in a storm. It helped save my wife and I more than once.

Today, Drew and Jessie are both doing well in college. They're living on their respective campuses and we could not be more proud. They keep in contact and support each other. We love having them home on school breaks because they're both so much fun to be around.

I like to think that part of the reason they're successful has to do with story time and mama laughs and poorly drawn ducks and the power of fun.

Because things are only as special as you make them.

50 BEING WHO YOU ARE

Lots of kids aren't happy being who they are.

Particularly if they have neurobiological conditions that make them tend to act different from other kids. Conditions like Asperger Syndrome, Higher Functioning Autism, Pervasive Developmental Disorder, Semantic-Pragmatic Disorder and others.

This can be hard on parents, too. When your child doesn't easily fit in, it's sometimes difficult to know when to keep him away from a situation that might make him feel worse about himself – or when it's best to keep him in a situation so he learns to deal with the world.

Being rejected is hard. That's when it's tempting for a kid to wish he was someone else – or at least wish he could be more like other kids. A new neighborhood, a new classroom, a new group of kids may seem like a chance to be someone else. He may think if he doesn't tell kids he meets about his condition, they won't notice.

Too often, of course, they notice – and tend to avoid him. Partly because they don't know the reason for his "different" behavior and don't know what they'd be getting into by associating with him.

So how can parents help bridge the gap?

By giving our kids reasons to be confident.

Confidence is magic. Have you ever noticed how people who are confident are social magnets? We tend to appreciate someone who is confident and who can demonstrate an ability we respect. Of course, being confident doesn't mean bragging or monopolizing a conversation. Projecting confidence without going overboard is an important social skill for our kids to learn.

Recently, I was looking through my high school yearbook. I was surprised when I came across one of my friend's pictures. Frankly, I remembered her as being a lot prettier. Then I realized, I'd confused being pretty with being attractive. She had a confident personality. She acted like she was attractive, so she was. There was much more to her than that yearbook picture could capture.

It was a lesson that we have some control over who we are. We can shape how other people perceive us by how we act towards them. Of course, learning to project confidence is not like learning to put on a coat. It's more like learning to play the piano. Not everyone can be a concert pianist, but anyone who works hard at practicing the piano is going to learn to play better.

Of course, our kids need things to be confident about, so we need to find and nurture their strengths. We also need to help them master everyday skills so they're comfortable dealing with real world situations.

When my son, Drew -- who has Asperger Syndrome -- was growing up, it was sometimes hard to know what he could learn to do on his own. My wife and I discovered a bit about self-fulfilling prophecies. When we acted worried that he couldn't learn something and continued to do it for him, he tended to let us. When we showed him we expected him do something on his own, he learned to do it, even if it took a while.

Every kid has different capabilities, of course, but isn't it devastating to think you may be holding your child back by being over-protective or underestimating him? Every kid fails a bit as he's learning.

I heard a self-help guru talk about teaching a child to walk. No little kid gets it on the first try. Or the second. Or the third. How would you respond if someone said to you at that point, "He's still falling down. I guess you'll have to carry him the rest of his life." You'd say, "No way! My kid is going to walk!" And you'd help him keep trying until he made it.

Like many other parents of kids with an autism spectrum disorder, I watched a recent episode of the TV show "Supernanny," in which the host brought in an autism expert (Lynn Kern Koegel, Ph.D) to help a family who has an autistic son.

The most important aspect of the program showed the parents learning that their autistic child was capable of far more than they'd imagined. Some of the training methods they learned were tough and didn't show immediate results. But in sticking with it, the family helped the three-year old boy with autism begin interacting positively and even start talking.

As parents, we all want to help our kids succeed, not make them overly dependent. The need to help our kids learn independence also applies to parents of kids without special needs. I saw learning expert Dr. Mel Levine on TV recently, talking about kids attending college today with unrealistic expectations. He said many have had their activities managed so heavily by their parents that they hadn't learned to plan and advocate for themselves. These kids expected to get good jobs right out of college and be granted quick promotions to exciting careers – without any special effort on their part. It was as if they assumed someone in the work world would take over their parents' role of watching out for them.

My son called his mom and me from college the other day and left a concerned message. He was missing some paperwork he needed to deal with the campus bureaucracy and make sure he got his first paycheck for his student job on campus -- and he wanted us to look for it and call him back.

We couldn't find what he needed, but we called back and left him a message, ready to offer advice on dealing with the situation.

When we finally connected, he'd found the paperwork in his dorm room, met with the person he needed to see and solved the problem on his own. That was a small victory in the grand scheme of things, but a great moment for us as parents.

It reminded me of other moments, like when Drew started buying things in stores by himself, after we helped him remember to focus on not getting distracted when standing in a checkout line and how to deal with the checkout clerk. It reminded me of him getting his driver's license after lots and lots of practice with us and a driving school instructor.

And there were times when what seemed like liabilities turned out to be assets in disguise. For example, Drew had real trouble writing in grade school. Forming letters was difficult for him. His sentences were tentative and awkward. It would have been easy to assume he just couldn't write. But we found it was actually a mechanical problem. Because Drew had trouble with his handwriting, he often lost his train of thought before he could capture it. When he began dictating his work, his sentences became increasingly sophisticated. Later, when he started working on a computer, keyboarding let him write freely on his own. Now he's an English major who's considering a career in technical writing and who's working on a novel.

Mastering everyday skills, being a good writer and being an expert in Japanese anime are just a few of the things that make Drew a lot more confident and happy now than he was when he was younger. He's hit some walls in getting to where he is today. But the experience has helped him learn to get over them or take another direction.

Having Asperger Syndrome is a part of who Drew is. He's confident enough to be open about it with anyone he feels needs to know. Among other things, this means he doesn't have to worry about his friends "finding out" and wondering if having AS was something he felt he had to conceal.

It's easy for a kid who's considered odd and who takes lots of hits to his self-esteem to want to hide why he's different. But if he can gain the confidence to help classmates see his differences for what they are -- and look past them to see his strengths -- he's taking a big step toward having people in his future appreciate him for who he is.

Sometimes you find that the person you really want to be is somewhere inside you. You just have to find a way to let him out.

###

Dan Coulter

51 EXPECTATIONS AND BEST DAYS

(Dan and Julie Coulter co-authored this article.)

What's your best day ever? We had one of our best days recently when our son, Drew, graduated from college. It's hard to describe just how big a deal this is for our family. Both of us went to college, and from the time we planned to have kids, we assumed they'd go to college, too.

But when we discovered Drew had Asperger Syndrome, all those plans got thrown up in the air. Actually, the plans went airborne a lot earlier, sometime after Drew got the first of a series of diagnoses starting in preschool when he had trouble socializing with other kids. By the time we got the AS diagnosis when he was fourteen, we'd had years to worry if he'd ever be able to leave home, much less go to college.

This was one of the things that ran through our heads as we sat in the commencement audience at St. Andrews Presbyterian College in Laurinburg, N.C. It was a warm spring day under a clear, Carolina-blue sky. After the ceremony, we shared our thoughts with each other.

St. Andrews is built on two sides of a lake, with the academic buildings on one side and the student center, dorms and athletic center on the other. Students cross the lake on a walking causeway bridge to get from their dorms to their classes.

The commencement would be held, appropriately, on the academic side. From the far side of the lake, we heard the faint sounds of bagpipes. We could just make out a double line of students in royal-blue caps and gowns, starting across the bridge.

We thought about Drew's early school days, when we kept hearing about how smart he was, but how isolated he was from most classmates. We thought about how we'd constantly had to adjust our expectations as he was growing up. We remembered the great support he'd had from so many teachers and other school staff. There were the elementary school teachers who understood when Drew's mom served as a stenographer to record his homework before he learned to type, because his brain moved faster than his awkward handwriting. There was the middle school teacher who put a small sofa in her room and told Drew that whenever he was over-stressed in her class or during lunch, he could sit on the sofa and take a break. Drew had a caring social worker in high school who helped arrange his class schedule with teachers who were understanding, guided him through tough times and celebrated his successes. Drew's chemistry teacher started an after-school role playing game club, allowing Drew — for the first time in high school — to form a group of friends he could hang out with.

The line of students was now half way across the causeway, led by a kilted bagpipe and drum band playing a stirring rendition of "Scotland The Brave." Along with other parents, we were on our feet with our video camera rolling. Drew came into view, looking sharp in his cap and gown.

We thought about how we'd had to find ways to help Drew expect a lot from himself and set high goals, without putting too much pressure on him. Helping Drew find ways to succeed gave him a sense of self-worth that counteracted the teasing and harassment he often experienced. During the summer before his junior year in high school, Drew played the wizard in "Once Upon A Mattress" at a college-sponsored theater workshop, throwing himself into the role and doing a stellar job. There's nothing quite like the boost applause gives you. Even though we weren't sure Drew could attend college, we encouraged him to take college prep classes and made modifications to his Individual Education Plan each year to encourage him to function independently. If college hadn't been right for Drew, that would have been fine. But we wanted to make sure we gave Drew the opportunity to go if it was right for him.

The soon-to-be graduates were now filing into their seats. Drew spotted us and flashed us a grin. For the umpteenth time, we looked at his name in the commencement booklet, marked by an asterisk that noted he was in the honors program.

We thought of how worried we were when we dropped him off at college as a freshman, eleven hours by car away from where we lived at the time. In spite of our concerns about having him get his assignments done without mom and dad to check up on him, he settled successfully into college life. St. Andrews is a relatively small school where Drew was able to thrive. He got to know his professors on an individual basis and made friends who shared his love of Japanese Anime and role-playing games. While there were bumps in the road, each year Drew met new challenges. His senior year, he got a job as a computer lab monitor and earned his own spending money. As a creative writing major, he worked feverishly to complete a screenplay and thesis during his last few months of college. His last semester's grades were his highest.

The speakers offered their advice and the graduates began crossing the stage. Drew accepted his diploma, then posed for a quick photo shaking hands with the college president. The ceremony ended with a recessional, accompanied again by the bagpipes and drums, and Drew was a college graduate.

You can look at this as a four-year accomplishment, but we see it as more of a 22-year accomplishment. Because of Asperger Syndrome, Drew often had to work twice as hard to accomplish half as much. He looked and spoke like a typical, bright kid in so many ways, it was hard for most people to understand why he also acted just a bit different. Why he couldn't just try harder to conform, as if that was a simple choice and not a continuous, frustrating struggle.

As the sound of the bagpipes died away, Drew met us, his sister and grandparents for big smiles, congratulations and hugs all round. Even though he was eager to seek out his college friends and tell them goodbye, he endured a round of family snapshots first with good humor. Later, at the graduates' reception, we met some of Drew's professors and heard their positive comments about him. Drew's creative writing professor gave him a book as a graduation present. Finally, we packed Drew's final few items, piled in our cars and headed home.

Of course, college graduation is more a beginning than an end. Drew's now faced with finding a job, living truly on his own -- not just independently in a college dorm -- and managing his life. He met his expectation to finish college — a goal that helped him graduate. Now he has to develop new expectations, not to mention dealing with his parents' expectations.

The lesson we all learned was to keep our expectations realistically high. To constantly change them to fit not just new situations, but new opportunities. To support expectations and make them not a source of anxiety and pressure, but a bridge.

Because these kinds of expectations can lead to some of your best days ever.

###

52 GENERATING GOOD SURPRISES

Damon Runyon, author of the play, "Guys and Dolls" once said, "The race is not always to the swift, nor the battle to the strong, but that's the way to bet."

Whatever races and battles you're dealing with, life is full of surprises.

If you're raising one or more children who are on the autism spectrum, you've probably had your fill of negative surprises. That's a given.

But the positive surprises can more than compensate for the negative, if we keep ourselves in the right frame of mind to take advantage of them.

I say, never take a positive surprise for granted. We have to be careful that training ourselves not to show disappointment doesn't also block us from showing appreciation and enthusiasm when our kids demonstrate something they've learned or accomplished. I think encouraging and then reinforcing positive behavior is one of the most powerful teaching tools we have.

Granted, teaching children who are on the spectrum can be a challenge, especially when you're dealing with brains that are not always naturally wired to understand the interactions and relationships most people take for granted.

My son Drew has Asperger Syndrome. He's highly capable in a number of areas. The other day I watched as he helped my wife resolve a complicated sales tax problem in the accounting for our business. Looking at her computer screen, the solution was obvious to him. But there have been plenty of times when I've wished that he was just as capable of sensing other people's feelings and needs.

With this in mind, I got a pleasant surprise the other day.

First, some quick background. Early in December, I had some shoulder surgery and spent about a month with my right arm in a sling. Even though I'm out of the sling now, I'm supposed to take it easy with the arm. During one of our family meetings, my wife, Julie, realized that she would be out of town on the day of my first physical therapy appointment. She suggested that Drew drive me. Drew volunteered to drop me at the clinic, do some shopping, and then pick me up. I agreed with Julie that I'd have Drew drive me if my arm didn't feel up to it. On the day of the appointment, however, I let Drew know that I'd drive myself.

When I emerged from my session of arm-stretching, I found Drew in the waiting room. We walked outside, and I asked him if he'd forgotten that I'd driven myself. He said, no, but while he was shopping, he got concerned that I might not feel up to driving home, so he'd stopped by just in case.

I was touched, and told him how much I appreciated his thoughtfulness.

His consideration reinforced the fact that difficulty in seeing the appropriate way to respond in a given situation doesn't necessarily mean that a person on the spectrum doesn't care or that he isn't trying hard to understand and do the right thing. Time after time, Drew has surprised us with bursts of development in areas that have been difficult for him.

If you're the parent of a younger child on the autism spectrum and you're working hard to help your child, but you're not always seeing a lot of progress, I'd like to offer an observation.

I can't guarantee that all the time and patience you invest now will make him or her swifter and stronger in the races and battles that matter the most in the future. Or that your efforts will help produce positive surprises along the way.

But that's the way to bet.

###

53 YOU DON'T HAVE TO GO IT ALONE

If you're raising a child with autism or Asperger syndrome, you don't have to go it alone.

I've met a lot of parents who are super-dedicated to their kids. Sometimes they feel they can only depend on themselves. This is more likely to happen if they run into roadblocks from schools, insurance companies or other organizations they had looked to for support.

Self reliance is important, but when dealing with the autism spectrum, I've seen overdoses of it result in anxiety, stress and burnout.

One way to avoid these problems is to continually look for new sources of support. I was recently involved in a recognition program that allowed me to learn about a lot of special individuals who've made life better for people with autism or Asperger Syndrome and their families.

Let me share a few examples:

A mom in Missouri was concerned that the male teacher her son had been assigned for the third grade might be intimidating for a child with Asperger Syndrome who'd previously only had female teachers. The teacher turned out to be sensitive and understanding and made her son feel safer than anyone he'd worked with before.

Many moms and dads in Eastern North Carolina are better off because of an autism advocate who works in a TEACCH center, facilitates support groups, trains police officers and camp counselors about autism and tours schools to advocate for better services for kids with special needs. She understands these needs all the better because she has a son with autism.

Hundreds of families in Arizona have received information about Asperger Syndrome and encouragement because a mother of a son with AS started an extensive support group in her state. Through her intensive volunteer efforts, both families with new diagnoses and "veterans" have a trusted community they can look to for support.

A mom in Sydney, Australia credits the teacher of a high-functioning autism class with transforming her son from a depressed and isolated child to one who looks forward to school and takes pride in his work. This mother marveled that the teacher took such a comprehensive approach, helping her son with timetables, organization, school work and social issues.

In New Jersey, a school principal helped a family learn to "let go" of anxiety about their son with Asperger Syndrome by providing an atmosphere where whatever happens during the school day is treated calmly, fairly and with dignity.

In Wisconsin, an autism spectrum disorders consultant helped a family see that previous advice focusing on negative consequences increased their son's sense of failure and isolation. By teaching the family about positive behavior supports and other helpful strategies, this consultant helped the son become more stable and social and focus on his talents and interests.

All of these families report dramatic improvements in their lives because of special people who provided them support. Some lucked into these encounters; others had to seek them out.

If your family hasn't found the help you feel you need, keep looking. Support groups can be great networking sources. Many experts in autism and Asperger Syndrome are willing to visit informally after lectures and seminars and offer direction. Experienced counselors may have ideas that we'd never think of ourselves.

The more we look, the greater the chances we'll find special people who can supercharge our lives for the better. Your family's supercharger may be just a day or a phone call away.

Good hunting!

###

54 THE DAY YOUR CHILD SAYS THANKS

I just sent off a Mother's Day package to my mom. As part of it, I found photos of myself at various ages (beginning with a baby picture) and scanned them into my computer to print onto her card.

Thinking about mom and looking at those pictures drove home to me what an empathetic, caring mom I've always had. I started to say "an extraordinary mom," but how can I make a comparison with other moms? And if other moms care just as much about their kids, that couldn't make my mom any less wonderful.

And she is wonderful. My mom dedicated her life to her kids. As I was growing up, she helped me in ways that I didn't, maybe couldn't, appreciate at the time.

This makes me think of all the moms I've talked with who struggle every day to help their kids with autism or Asperger Syndrome. Many are concerned because their sons and daughters don't demonstrate a lot of empathy for others, including mom. It can be hard to pour your heart and soul into a child and not see appreciation in his eyes or hear it in her voice.

My son with Asperger Syndrome, Drew, is now 24 years old. Last night after eating, he hugged his mom, kissed her on the cheek and said, "Wonderful dinner, mom." This sort of spontaneous appreciation is common for him now — and would have been hard to imagine when he was ten, or even fifteen, years old. Of course, a lack of appreciation through your teenage years isn't unique to kids on the autism spectrum. Lots of parents of typically developing kids can testify to that.

But expressing appreciation can be an extra challenge to kids on the spectrum because they're dealing with developmental delays. The good news: what they don't understand today, they may be able to understand in the future. My wife, Julie, is as special to my son as my mother is to me. And Julie glows each time Drew expresses the appreciation he didn't show only a few years ago. The turning point came after he graduated from high school.

As he made more friends, he encountered some who came from families where impatience and criticism were common, and acceptance and positive reinforcement were rare. That's when he came home and thanked us for the way he was raised.

No one can make guarantees, but the more you give, the more likely you are to get the feedback dedicated moms deserve. If you have a young child or teenager on the spectrum and your family is anything like ours, you have a lot to look forward to. Reaching the day when your child's eyes are opened to what you truly gave him, and he reaches out to you, is a feeling like no other.

55 TURNING FAILURE INTO SUCCESS IN THE FOURTH DIMENSION

Ever gotten frustrated when you've failed? I have. It's especially hard when you feel that you're somehow failing as a parent – or that your child is failing at something and you can't fix the problem.

If you're trying hard and you've made repeated attempts, it can be especially disheartening.

But even this kind of failure can be a step toward success.

To illustrate, let's look at the movie, "Back to the Future." Marty McFly, the time-traveling lead character, is a young musician who won't send his audition tape to a record company because he's afraid of failure. During the film, Marty is continually admonished by time machine inventor Doc Brown, "You're not thinking fourth dimensionally!" By that, he means Marty isn't taking the effects of time into account.

What does time and thinking fourth dimensionally have to do with failure and success?

Failure can feel final in the moment when you experience it. But it's really only final for that moment. The next moment, you can start looking for another way to succeed.

In the film, Doc Brown has a framed photo of Thomas Edison over his fireplace. Edison tried thousands of experiments that failed before finding a good filament for the first practical electric light blub. The inventor said of these failures, "They taught something that I didn't know. They taught me what direction to move in."

So, we just have to get into that mindset, right? Simple. Okay, not simple. But possible.

Late in the movie, we learn that Marty has what it takes to be a successful musician when he plays a knock-em-dead version of Johnny B. Goode on guitar at a high school dance. This means, like almost all other good musicians, Marty had learned to practice through his initial failures to play songs adeptly, gradually becoming better.

Just like off-key notes are part of learning to play a piano or guitar, failure is part of the process in raising children. And no matter how experienced you get, no one gets it perfect.

My kids are 23 and 24 years old. They're both doing well. But I still have moments when I wish I could convince each to do things differently – and fail. But I'm much less likely to let frustration hamper me than I used to be.

I've learned to be more strategic, and try less direct approaches.

For example, when you encounter a behavior you want to change, biting your tongue and not commenting may be the best way to start the change process.

Let's say you're at dinner with your family and your daughter is taking large bites of food and talking with her mouth full. It's tempting to correct her then and there. But if you've tried that before and it just caused an emotional scene, maybe it's better to let it go for the moment. Then, plan a session where you sit with her and talk about it. Be inventive. Who are her favorite movie stars? Maybe you could find a movie that involves one of them sitting at a dinner table eating with good manners. Show her that section of the video and practice eating a meal with just you and her. Describe how you are both going to eat beforehand, demonstrate doing it right, then let her try. Make it fun. Don't expect too great a change in one session. Eat a number of private, practice meals. Talk about the benefits of eating politely. Praise progress.

Generating even a small success can help your child feel, well, successful. And success is a great building block to more success. Especially if you take on behaviors you want to change one at a time.

At the end of the movie, Marty (having traveled to the past, overcome numerous failures, and helped his father find new ways to succeed) returns to the future to find things changed for the better. He also finds a new optimism.

The lesson is that success or failure can be a state of mind. If you're willing to use patience and keep trying new approaches, you can always be in the process of turning failure into success where it counts -- fourth dimensionally.

###

IMPROVING FAMILY LIFE

56 STACKING THE DECK FOR FAMILY HOLIDAYS

It's family holiday gatherings season.

So, do you feel anticipation or anxiety?

If you have a child with an autism spectrum disorder, you might feel a bit of both.

My wife and I are veterans of years of extended family gatherings with our son who has Asperger Syndrome. We've learned that the proper preparation is a great insurance policy toward making the gathering a positive experience for everyone.

First, size up the situation realistically. What will your family event be like? How is your son or daughter with an ASD likely to react in that environment? What can you do to influence the environment and prepare your child?

Let's say you have a son named Bill who has Asperger Syndrome.

If you're going to be seeing family who doesn't often interact with Bill, consider writing a letter or email to those who will attend. Tell them you want to help ensure that everyone has a good time, so you want to explain that, because Bill has Asperger Syndrome, he may act or react a bit differently than they're used to.

The letter should be positive. It should not tell people how they have to act to accommodate Bill. It should focus on the nice experience everyone can have if family members make some adjustments to help Bill fit in.

For example, Bill loves studying weather, has learned a lot about weather, and is always eager to talk about weather. You can write that it would be great if you could work with the others who will attend the gathering to plan some games or activities or decorations that relate to weather. And explain that if Bill goes on a bit too long about weather, it's O.K. to say, "I'm really impressed with all you know about weather, Bill, but I'm not as interested in it as you are, and I'd like to talk about something else now."

The key is to help others understand how Bill is likely to act and react, and give them suggestions on interacting with Bill that will help keep things positive. If Bill is likely to exhibit behaviors that could be interpreted as rude or tactless, explain that he doesn't mean to offend, it's just the way his brain processes information. Be honest, but upbeat. Ask parents to share appropriate information about being patient with Bill with their children.

Consider past experience to determine how closely you, or someone else who knows what to expect, needs to supervise Bill in this environment. You may need to limit your stay or identify a quiet place where Bill can be by himself with a book or a game or a DVD if the situation becomes overwhelming for him.

In your letter, you can also inquire about the other children who will attend and ask if there's anything special the group might plan or do for them. After all, you want the visit to be special for everyone.

Finally, talk with Bill about what to expect and help him practice the social skills you want him to use. The more Bill knows about the gathering in advance and how to deal with it, the more confident and comfortable he's likely to be.

You might choose to write a social story describing the upcoming event. My wife once wrote a "news story" about our niece's wedding and read it to our son in the car as we traveled to another state for the ceremony. Consider your child's history as you plan your briefing. You may decide to provide less detail if your child is very literal minded and gets upset when things don't turn out exactly the way he or she expects they will.

A lot of families (ours included) have attended events simply hoping for the best. But we've learned that hope is more realistic if you stack the deck. Where extended family gatherings are concerned, you may need to mark it, stack it, and stick a few cards up your sleeve.

But everybody wins.

###

57 GRANDPARENT POWER!

The word "family" can evoke powerful memories and emotions. Thinking of family recalls the Robert Frost line, "Home is the place where, when you have to go there, they have to take you in." When grandparents are involved, the line could often be changed to, "…they can't wait to take you in."

The relationships between kids and their grandparents can provide some of the strongest extended family ties. When families have children on the autism spectrum, these ties can be a tremendous resource for both the kids and their parents. Of course, that resource works best when parents and grandparents cooperate closely.

I remember a shopping trip with my grandfather early in elementary school. We lived in Maryland and my mom's folks had taken the train from Missouri for a rare visit. It was magical to be with these wonderfully attentive folks who I only really knew from stories and pictures. My grandfather took me to the store to buy some school supplies, including crayons. The list in his hand called for a pack of twelve colors. But, being a grandparent, he bought me the box of 64. When we got home, my mom laughed and say said, "Oh, daddy, you didn't have to buy that big box! The smaller box would have been fine."

It was a small substitution that didn't cause any problems and also made me happy, so this "grandparent indulgence" was no problem. For a child on the spectrum, however, having grandparents who act in accordance with a parent's directions and approach -- sometimes even on small things -- can be extremely important. Consistency is often an obsession for kids on the spectrum and they can have rigid likes and dislikes. If you don't know your grandchild really well, you could be stunned when buying the "wrong" flavor of ice cream sends a smiling child into a sudden emotional meltdown.

Tried and true parenting techniques that work fine with your other grandkids may just not work with autistic children. Also, each child with autism is an individual, so parents often have to go to great lengths to determine what works best for their child. The brains of kids with autism are wired a bit differently, so even if they're on the higher-functioning end of the spectrum, with a condition such as Asperger Syndrome, some things that are easy for other kids can be tough for them. For example, many have a difficult time learning and applying social skills. Parents often have to pick out the most important behaviors to work on and let the less important ones slide.

As grandparents, you don't want to be too quick to make judgments about parents' actions when you may only see part of a very complicated situation. Did you ever get frustrated with your parents because they criticized your actions based on only part of the picture?

If you're a grandparent of a child on the spectrum and you're close to the family and providing lots of support, bless your heart! You're probably already tuned in to what we're talking about here. If you're a grandparent who's been separated by distance or other factors and you'd like to be closer, here are some steps you can take to build bonds with your grandkids.

Talk with your son or daughter and his or her spouse about your grandchild. Find out as much as you can about the child's condition and what they're doing to help and support him or her. Ask how you can help and how they want you to deal with any challenging behaviors. Kids with autism often face a lot of rejection, so some of the most important things you can offer are love, patience, and unconditional acceptance. This comes more naturally to some grandparents than to others, but it can mean a lot to a child who others may see simply in terms of his or her problems.

People often focus on the problems of autism, but there's another side to the story. You may find that spending time with an autistic grandchild lets you be with a fun person who just looks at the world a bit differently. Sometimes letting go of what a child might have been helps you truly appreciate who he is. My son, who has Asperger Syndrome, has a great relationship with his grandparents, who live nine hours away, but visit frequently. He's also lucky to have relatives who live close by, including a great-uncle who always enjoys swapping jokes whenever they're together.

It's important to recognize that kids on the spectrum often have significant strengths as well as challenges. You may be the person who can help draw out those strengths and help your grandchild prepare to deal as independently as possible with the outside world. What a feeling it is to make a real, positive difference in a child's life.

Spending time with your grandkids can help build a relationship that gives parents the confidence to leave a child who needs special attention in your care. It can be hard to find spectrum-savvy baby sitters, so perhaps you can enable stressed-out parents to go out for some much-needed, worry-free recreation.

Sometimes, parents just need someone to listen. Lending your ear may help them put things in perspective. If you have advice to offer (you do, don't you?), it's more likely to be taken if you use the recipe of ten parts listening to one part advice. Also, make sure you know what you're talking about and focus on the benefits of what you're suggesting. Be aware that it's common for parents of kids on the spectrum to be wary of unsolicited advice, particularly if they've heard people routinely suggest therapies that don't apply, or make simplistic observations like, "He just needs more discipline." Even if you have good advice to give, you may have to overcome "advice burnout."

The best way to have your counsel taken is to really listen to the parents, really do your research and, hopefully, spend enough time with the child that you show his or her parents you really understand the situation. Always focus on the benefits of what you're suggesting. If you still sense resistance, you might try approaching the subject by asking questions. "I read about treatment 'XYZ' where children responded well. Is that something that you think might help Jimmy?"

I've seen some situations where one or both parents were in denial about a child's condition, and the grandparents diplomatically encouraged the parents to have the child tested or to seek support. This encouragement can be a tremendous benefit to the parents and grandchild.

With some parents, however, it's a challenge to help them see through their denial. If you push too hard, you risk having them throw up a wall that keeps you from helping your grandkids. Just remember that sometimes parents are mourning the loss of the child they expected your grandson or granddaughter to be. Again, patience and a lot of listening is a good strategy to put you in a position to influence the situation in a positive way.

I also know of situations where grandparents are actually raising their grandkids. It's a special kind of caring when "extended family" becomes just "family" because that's what children need.

Even though grandparents have the full range of strengths and flaws that we all have, that special connection with grandkids often seems to bring out the best in people. Ideally, grandparents have just enough distance to see things realistically, are close enough to really care, and have the experience to be effective.

But caring counts most. When I think of my own grandparents, I realize that my best memories are not about the size of the crayon box granddad bought me. They're about special people caring a whole lot about making my life colorful and fun. They made me look forward to every minute I was with them.

What better gift could you give?

58 FAMILY

Who's in your family?

It may be larger than you think.

My wife, Julie, and I recently went to her annual "Johnson family reunion." We showed a video there that we'd produced about several generations of family history using interviews and old photographs. We included a story about great-grandfather Rommie trying to drive his new Model T Ford for the first time. When it abruptly started forward and he couldn't remember how to stop it, he clung to the steering wheel yelling, "Whoa! Gee! Gee! Haw!" as if he was driving one of his mules. His oldest son jumped up on the car's running board and got it stopped.

The older members of Julie's family grew up together. As children, her father and his cousins spent their summers together working on family members' farms. They love telling tales about the work, play and shenanigans they shared. It makes some of them wistful when younger members of the family, who didn't grow up with their cousins and don't feel the same sense of kinship, don't put as high a priority on attending family reunions.

This is probably an inevitable result of a mobile population, in which extended families can live great distances away and rarely see each other. The older members of my wife's family are close because they understand one another. They speak the same language. And they're always ready to help and support each other.

If you're lucky enough to be close to your extended kinfolk, that's great. But you don't have to be related to people to feel a sense of family. Parents with children who have special needs such as Asperger Syndrome or autism can feel very alone. Especially if their extended family lives far away and may not recognize what they're dealing with on a daily basis.

This is when contact with others dealing with similar situations can be a lifesaver.

Like the mother I know of who rescued another mother taking her developmentally delayed autistic son to a "Thomas the Tank Engine" exhibit at a transportation museum.

In the museum's gift shop, 11 year old, 150 pound Aaron flopped down on the floor and threw a tantrum in the midst of the other, mostly two and three year-old, Thomas fans.

Desperately trying to deal with the situation and purchase the new "Thomas" DVD her son had picked out, Aaron's mom, Lynn, felt someone grab her shoulder. She thought to herself, "If you say one word I'll…!"

But she turned to find a woman who said, "Give me your stuff and give me your money and I'll pay for it. I'll meet you in the parking lot. I have a son with autism."

Lynn managed, with a struggle, to get her son to her car. A short while later, the woman and her daughter appeared to deliver the DVD and Lynn's change. The rescuer gave Lynn a hug and said, "Sometimes this is all we can do."

Then the daughter said, "You should have seen my mom."

"What did she do?"

"The security guard was having a problem and said 'they shouldn't let kids like that in places like this.' And she looked him straight in the eye and said 'If you've got a typical child, you go home tonight and pray to God you never have to go through anything like this'!"

Lynn said it touched her deeply that someone else knew what she was going through.

Those of us with children on the autism spectrum are sometimes in the best position to give each other the help and support we need. We know what it feels like. We speak each other's language.

We're family.

###

TAPPING A MOTHER'S STRENGTH

59 ASPERGER SYNDROME AND MOM'S SECRET WEAPON

This is for all the moms of children with Asperger Syndrome.

Want to be more effective in helping your child? Want to give him the best possible training to deal with AS and succeed? Then you need to access a secret weapon.

You.

Your immediate reaction may be, "Yeah, right! I'm already doing everything I can. More than I can! In fact, I'm so stressed that just the thought of doing more threatens to shut me down."

But I bet you're overlooking something. Over the years since our son was diagnosed, I've talked with a lot of mothers of kids with AS. And I've watched my wife, who, like most AS moms, has taken on the main burden of researching AS and dealing with schools, doctors and on and on and on. A common thread that ties many of these moms together is frustration. Look at AS online discussion boards and see how often moms talk about failing and being discouraged day after day.

But how many are truly failing? I think these moms care so passionately about their kids and want them to succeed so badly that they don't give themselves enough credit for what they're accomplishing.

If you have a goal for your child and you don't reach that goal, do you give yourself credit for the progress you helped your child make toward that goal? If you try your hardest to reach the top of a mountain and you make it halfway up, did you fail? YOU MADE IT HALFWAY UP A MOUNTAIN! And maybe you established a base camp to help you reach the top in the future.

Like many AS moms I've met, my wife easily qualifies for sainthood. Over the years, she's worked closely with our son, Drew, and with teachers and principals and psychologists and support groups and more. Drew is now living three hours away from us in college. He's making good grades and has friends. And my wife still frets over the messy state of his dorm room and worries she should have gotten him more "executive function" training.

My point is that no matter how much or how little progress you make, it's easy to overlook that progress and focus on falling short of perfection. My wife told me about hearing a psychologist warn, "Don't 'should' on yourself." That's always obsessing: "I should have done this," or "If I'd only done that."

Focusing on failure is depressing. It robs you of energy and generates stress. On the other hand, don't you feel good when you succeed? Don't you feel energized and optimistic? Don't you have better ideas and relate better to people?

That's the secret weapon. And you can legitimately tap into it if you just break down your objectives and goals into steps and give yourself credit for every step you and your child make toward success.

I've seen the results with kids. Praise their progress and they work harder to reach a goal. Criticize them and they tend to shut down and avoid even trying. The same thing works for us. If you focus on feeling good about progress instead of criticizing yourself for failure, your secret weapon kicks in.

Don't get me wrong. I'm not saying set low goals and be happy with mediocrity. I'm saying that giving yourself legitimate credit can put you into a positive frame of mind that gives you energy and better ideas. And if you have a positive attitude and energy when "Plan A" falls short, you're more likely to try "Plan B" -- and "Plan C" and "Plan D." My son has already exceeded expectations so many times I can't count them. In big ways and in small ways. And if I've played a significant part, it's because my wife helped me see the role I needed to play.

Them wives are heaven-sent.

So set your goals high. Help your child find the best in himself. Help her find the best in others. Don't settle for less than your best. But you may be the only person in a position to truly appreciate all you're doing for your child. So step back occasionally. Look at the progress you've made in the face of pretty stiff obstacles. And give yourself a pat on the back.

I'm betting you deserve a lot more than that -- and I hope you see your reward in the eyes of your child every Mother's Day for the rest of your life.

###

60 FEEDBACK FOR MOTHERS

We all want to make a difference. We all crave feedback.

As Mothers' Day gets closer, I'm thinking about moms of kids with Asperger Syndrome and other Autism Spectrum Disorders who give a lot, but don't always get a lot of feedback from their kids. The way their kids' brains are wired sometimes makes it hard for them to express appreciation -- or let mom know how much impact she's having.

But so many mothers keep up the support, constantly working with their kids to help them overcome their frustrations and make the most of their strengths. Some of these moms see breakthroughs in younger children. Some watch for years for confirmation that they're doing the right things and making a difference in their kids' lives. This applies to dads too. We'll talk about dads closer to Fathers' Day, but today's article is for moms.

Sometimes mothering is a shifting balance between joy and worry. If you're feeling like, "I've had my allotment of worry and would like a generous helping of joy, thank you very much," I'd like to share a moment my wife, Julie, had recently. Our son, Drew, who has Asperger Syndrome, has given his mom and me a lot of joy over the years. But this was a first.

Julie was on the phone with Drew, who's away at college. After they hung up, she turned to me and said, "Wow. For the first time in 21 years, Drew told me he loved me without me saying it first."

This made me think about the young man Drew's become and all the positive things I see in him that have been influenced by his mom.

A song Bette Midler sings called, "My Mother's Eyes," came to mind. The song was written by Tom Jans and it captures something about the lifelong bond between a mother and child. Jans writes about how he "got my mother's eyes" and about how the way he looks at the world was shaped by his mom.

Part of the song goes,
> "Well I keep walking with my head held high,
> with my head to the sky,
> with my mother's eyes."

Moms can give us our confidence and our conscience. My mom and dad were shaped the Great Depression and World War II. They always put their kids' needs first. At one time, my dad worked at three jobs (one full-time and two part-time) to provide for us. My mom was always there to make us feel safe and warm. She could tell great stories and defuse her kids' arguments with her sense of humor. Later in life, she did an amazing job of taking care of my dad before he passed away.

I still see right and wrong through the things she taught us kids and the example she set. I know I didn't express anywhere near enough appreciation while I was growing up. But I always felt special when Mom showed she was proud of me. (And Mom, because I know you'll read this, I still care about making you proud.)

Jans' song continues,
"Have I seen all that I could?
Have I seen more than I should?
With my mother's eyes?"

Your kids may not always let you know how much progress you're making, molding them into the best people they can be. They may not know themselves. But everything you do is helping to shape them and their values and give them at least some of the keys you've found to unlock a complicated world.

Whether or not you get direct feedback, I'm betting as you watch them grow, you'll see how much farther they go than they could have gone without you. And, as Julie and I learned, you never know when you'll get a burst of feedback about how much your guidance mattered. Is it possible to overestimate the influence a mother can have?

I know it would be hard to find a better measure for my most important decisions than how they'd look -- in my mother's eyes.

###

61 MOTHERS AND BELIEF

I finally went through a box of papers I got from my mom a while back, before she moved into a retirement home. It was a Dan shrine. I found every issue of the high school newspaper I edited. And mementos of every accomplishment or award she could get her hands on and save. Right down to a red ribbon I got for coming in second place in a sack race at church camp when I was in grade school. I called Mom and got her standard greeting, "How are you, honey? Is everyone feeling okay?"

I think every mom worries about her kids. But if my mom ever had a doubt about my worth or my ability to succeed in the world, I never saw it. There were plenty of times I doubted myself while I was growing up, but seeing my mom's confidence in me was a great antidote.

And if she had doubts, but mastered them so I couldn't see them, I think I appreciate that even more.

Many moms of children with Asperger Syndrome and autism have doubts thrust upon them. Sometimes by supposed experts who tell them what not to expect of their sons and daughters.

I thought of this when I heard an interview recently with Quinn Bradlee, a young man who has Velo-Cardio-Facial Syndrome. VCFS is not autism, but like autism, it can generate a range of physical problems and learning disabilities.

Quinn's mother, writer Sally Quinn, says she was told by a psychologist when her son was young that he would never lead a normal life and should be institutionalized. She and her husband, former Washington Post editor Ben Bradlee, refused. Quinn says his mother was his leading advocate and calls her a lioness for the way she always believed in him and fought for him.

While he's had a rough road, Quinn Bradlee is now 26. His accomplishments include writing a memoir, A Different Life: Growing Up Learning Disabled and Other Adventures, participating in a documentary about VCFS, and starting a website for people with learning disabilities: FriendsOfQuinn.com. He's recently made appearances on a number of national news programs, sometimes with his parents.

In an interview on PBS' News Hour, Sally Quinn explained her approach, "I think the most important thing is to love your child…and make them believe in themselves…there's a thing that the shrinks call 'mirroring,' when somebody looks in your eyes and they see themselves through your eyes. And I wanted always when Quinn looked in my eyes that he saw nothing but love, and appreciation and belief in him."

In our work with families dealing with Asperger Syndrome and autism, my wife and I see more and more parents taking this positive approach. Refusing to accept that their children can't do something without giving them an opportunity to try. Realizing that a child who believes he can accomplish a task is more likely to keep trying until he finds a way.

Society's view is changing, too, as children who once would have been written off are blowing past expectations. This is due, in no small part, to mothers.

Society is relearning an age-old lesson.

You don't mess with a lioness.

###

Life in the Asperger Lane

BECOMING ROLE MODEL FATHERS

62 BECOMING DAD THE INCOMPRABLE (A FATHERS DAY REFLECTION)

I was awake most of the night last night — lying in bed thinking about being a dad. And thinking about two truths: It's tough being a dad. It's great being a dad.

It's easy to get caught up in the first truth, especially if you have a child with problems or special needs. But the second truth is where all the fun is – and where you find the power to be the father your kids want and need.

The first truth is never going to go away. But when you focus on it, spending time with your kids is an obligation. The second truth is more powerful. It's what you feel after the birth of your child. It's what you know when you look at that tiny face and see all the positive possibilities. It's what you understand when you first make your baby laugh.

We all have ups and downs as dads. But if you could, wouldn't you lock yourself in the great moments? The times when your kids think you're the best dad in the world? Dad the Incomparable, Lord High Protector and Benevolent Fun Machine! The guy who gets mobbed by a blur of childish joy when he hits the door and hears, "Daddy!!!"

I found a way. Look at a picture.

Yes. It's that simple.

Go around the house and search through the pictures you have of your child. Check the photo box in the closet. Find one that freezes time and brings back everything you felt and promised him when he was a baby; when she was a toddler. If there's more than one of your kids in the picture, or you have a picture of each, that's great.

Put the picture you choose in your wallet or a plastic protector. Take out the picture and look at it once an hour. Everyday.

It puts things in perspective. It can help you hold your daughter's face in your mind to ease tense times at work. It can make you eager to get home to spend time with your son. It can make you more patient when you're dealing with your kids and help you really listen when they talk.

It can help you stop and think before you criticize your son, "Is this the way I want him to remember me the rest of his life?" The small picture in your wallet can help you see the big picture. If you treat every contact with your child as one that might stand out in his mind as he grows up, will you treat him differently? The picture can help you do things the way you really want to do them anyway -- and make your kids want to always try their hardest to make their dad proud.

It usually takes something big to change our lives. But sometimes, we can change our own lives with little things, like looking at a picture.

###

63 WHAT'S A DAD WORTH?

I heard a discussion about a dad's worth the other day as I was radio channel surfing in my car. Two talk show hosts were hotly debating some comments made by actress Nicole Kidman. The topic: does a rich single mom have anything to complain about? The female host said that even a famous, wealthy single mom can have it tough raising kids. The macho male host wasn't buying it. "Come on, she's got jillions of dollars! She can buy anything she needs."

He might have been more persuasive if he'd pointed out that many divorced dads are devoted to their kids and not all single moms are raising kids alone. But the argument that you could buy what a dad does makes this guy sound pretty clueless.

Or maybe it says something sad about his relationship with his father.

A dad who shows his kids he cares about them can be one of the most powerful influences in their lives. This is especially true of kids with special challenges, such as Asperger Syndrome.

Dads are incredible role models. Who hasn't been proud -- or mortified -- to see your child copy something you do? You're teaching even when you're not trying. And dads who put real effort into raising their kids get the biggest rewards.

I think the dads who have the most impact are the ones who find ways to really enjoy being with their kids - even kids with problems. From the other side of the picture, kids who enjoy being with their dads are much more eager to listen to them and to try and make their dads proud as they grow up.

Here are a few things I've seen great dads do that can't be bought.

First, these dads let their faces light up every time they see their child and show him it's a treat to see him. This makes a son or daughter feel really special - like an injection of self-worth. And there's nothing like self-worth to combat negative influences outside your home. If your child feels great being with you, doing things together is more like recreation than obligation. As a bonus, you're likely to wind up having more fun and finding ways to spend more time with your kids.

Second, these dads kick into "patient gear" whenever they deal with their kids. It's easy to forget that talking isn't teaching and hearing something once doesn't mean a kid understands and the ins and outs of what you're talking about. Taking the time to understand how much your child is absorbing of what you're saying can really help him learn. Some kids don't pick up social skills intuitively, just by observing others. If this is your child, you have to figure out how to help him understand. As a dad, you need to be like the test pilots in Tom Wolfe's book, "The Right Stuff." If a test pilot's plane didn't perform as predicted and the normal procedures didn't work, he'd try something new, and something else new, and something else, until he found something that worked. You can do the same thing and you don't even need to worry about a parachute.

Third, these dads use consistent, measured discipline and lots of positive reinforcement. Even if their child throws a tantrum in public, they don't let embarrassment tempt them into overreacting verbally or physically. Who doesn't respect a dad who is calm and patient with a child having a meltdown? Who hasn't seen a child glow from a dad's compliments? These dads teach a child what it means to be fair - and how to get the best out of people with praise.

Fourth, these dads look at things from their kids' point of view. They see that kids don't always understand when dad's had a hard day. These dads learn to leave problems at the door and let good times with their families bring up their spirits.

These are the dads I admire and try to be like.

The bottom line: every contact with your son or daughter is an opportunity. The way they feel about you the rest of their lives depends on the countless little interactions between the two of you every day. If you treat every contact with your child as one he could remember forever, you'll be the dad you really want to be.

That can't be measured in dollars. And, as a dad, it's kind of nice to know you're priceless.

###

64 DAD VERSION 2.0

I just had a great Father's Day. At one point, enjoying the day with my family, I considered how a dad's role has changed as my kids have grown older. I think a lot of dads are getting better.

I see more and more dads who are taking a larger role in their kids' lives, especially dads of children with special needs. Fewer dads who bury themselves in work and tell themselves that their contribution is to make a living for the family. More dads who share homework help and school meetings and doctor visits with moms.

Of course, some dads have always been full partners in raising kids. Some dads are raising kids alone and doing an incredible job. But many of us, myself included, have had to upgrade our concept of a dad's responsibilities. Especially those of us who had very traditional "Dad Version 1.0" role models.

It can be a rocky transition to "Dad 2.0". When you take on a new role, it's like starting a new job. You don't know all the ropes and you can make mistakes. If you're used to excelling at your previous jobs, it can be frustrating to make what seem like bone-headed parenting bloopers.

But it's all part of the process. It helps to remind yourself that nobody gets it perfect. Babe Ruth's baseball career batting average was .342. Hank Aaron's was .305. Two of the most celebrated sluggers who ever played the game succeeded in hitting the ball less than half the times they came to bat.

To take the baseball analogy a little further, it's always a good idea to do some scouting. Observe your kids. Figure out what motivates them and use what you learn to make the time you spend with them a better experience for everyone. Moms usually make great scouts. You can get probably get all sorts of positive information from a mom about your kids if you just ask. You might also take some batting practice. Think through what you're going to say to your kids before you say it and consider how they might react.

I've mentioned before that my wife and I are working on two videos to help siblings understand their brothers and sisters who have autism or

Asperger Syndrome. Some of the dads we interviewed for these programs are real Dad 2.0 role models.

One talks about a support group he's started for fathers of kids who have Asperger Syndrome.

A compassionate step-father describes working hard to help his neurotypical step-daughter understand that the family sometimes can't give her what she wants because they're committing resources toward giving their autistic daughter what she needs.

A dad whose autistic son has severe meltdowns explains how he tries to see things from his son's point of view to give him insights to help calm things down.

A father who describes his wife as "the main caregiver" urges dads to stay home and spend "daddy time" with the kids, while giving mom a regular night out with her friends. He also recommends not being afraid to try things that haven't worked in the past, noting that his autistic son has now learned to behave in restaurants after a long period when the family had just stopped eating out.

A dad with both autistic and neurotypical sons advises, "You have to live in the present and pray for the future…you have to live life to the fullest like anyone else. You cannot allow autism to lock you up in a box."

Showing our kids we care and pushing ourselves out of our comfort zones is all part of being a good dad, especially if you have kids with special needs. It's a way to ensure you don't miss any "Dad 2.0.1" or "Dad 2.0.2" updates, and prepare to be absolutely compatible with that "Dad 3.0" upgrade that's bound to come.

You might even be the one who writes the code.

###

65 A GPS FOR FATHERS DAY

Father's day is a celebration of the times we get it right.

The times we're wise and strong and patient, like the fathers in the 1950's sitcoms "Father Knows Best" and "Leave it to Beaver."

And that's great, because the more we get credit for the things we do that work, the more likely we are to repeat them.

Being a dad is a special challenge for fathers of children with Asperger Syndrome. You have to deal with all the normal parenting stuff, plus all the "Asperger Stuff." Frankly, it feels good when someone acknowledges what we're doing right.

Remember that first big step in becoming the father your child with Asperger Syndrome needs? When you realized that the conventional wisdom passed down by those sitcom fathers often doesn't work with the Asperger Stuff. Because their advice maps were laid out by people who'd never navigated the intricacies of AS. Frankly, some of the directions in those maps don't work that well with typical kids, including, "You just have to stand up to bullies." When you try that road with our children, it leads to disaster.

But we learn.

We learn to draw our own maps, based on what we discover on mental excursions with our highly individual offspring.

Somewhere along the way, we stop to think how much our happiness depends on making our families happy. Hearing your children laugh and getting a thank you hug is addictive. These responses can be harder to spark in a child with AS, but that makes success even sweeter.

Teaching our children is partly about learning that short cuts rarely work. Success usually requires taking the longer road of explaining things in terms that make sense in the unique universe behind those skeptical eyes.

I really appreciate those fathers who make the extra effort to interact with other dads and pool what they've learned. I know of one such dad in Charlotte, North Carolina, who started a local support group for fathers of children with AS.

I think such support groups are great. About ten years ago, when we lived in Atlanta, the minister of the church we attended saw how isolated men could become, busy with their jobs and families. He held an event where a bunch of men in the church got together, broke into groups of six or so, and told their life stories. My group of busy dads decided to make time to meet on Saturday mornings for breakfast at a local restaurant. There was no agenda. We talked about whatever was on our minds. At first, mostly sports, yards, and work. And when we grew more comfortable, about family stuff. Comparing notes on which paths led to dead ends and which got us through the woods.

Justly or unjustly, dads are famous for not wanting to ask for directions.

But even if you just listen, getting together with other dads is like tapping into a database-packed GPS to help you figure out the right route to helping your child with Asperger Syndrome be successful and happy.

So take credit for your progress this Fathers Day. And think about whether that GPS could make the trip to your next Dad's Day even better.

###

Life in the Asperger Lane

HELPING SIBLINGS UNDERSTAND

66 AUTISM, ASPERGER SYNDROME AND SIBLINGS

During the past seven months, my wife and I have met an amazing group of people.

In producing two videos about brothers and sisters of kids on the autism spectrum, we've conducted 57 interviews with siblings and parents.

People were incredibly open about their lives. About their hopes, fears, and challenges. Most of all, about the ways they've found to make things better for their families. We went into these videos looking for "best practices" about siblings that we could share with other families. We got that and more.

Working on these programs has kept me from writing articles as often as I'd like, so I thought I'd take a break from editing and share a few comments from our interviews.

One of the videos covers the autism spectrum and the other focuses on Asperger Syndrome. The programs are divided into segments to appeal to siblings of different ages. These quotes are from the autism program's segment for seven to eleven year olds, which I happen to be working on today.

Let's start with Alex, a wonderfully patient eight year old whose younger twin sisters with autism used to bite the tails off his dinosaurs and stomp on his Lego space ship, until he learned to put his toys away where his sisters couldn't find them:

"Sometimes when we go in the car, I have to watch my sisters' movies, and it's Barney, Wiggles or Teletubbies, …really little kid shows…but I have to watch it…because that's what you have to do when you have autistic sisters or brothers."

"Sometimes my sisters cry at restaurants so my mom or dad has to take them out to the car, but if they keep crying, sometimes we have to leave. So don't get mad at that if they do that, because it's still just natural, because they haven't learned how to behave very well."

"My sisters learn to do things from me because they watch me. Like when I brush my teeth, they usually find a little toothbrush and they use it and they try to do it and it's making their teeth clean because they're starting to brush their teeth more often…"

"When Elizabeth and I are on the trampoline, we usually like to jump in the middle, but I like to bounce her…and she goes to the side and I bounce her and she laughs even more…and Emily likes that, too."

"Emily and Elizabeth have begun to ask me for help when they can't get anything or need to know how to get it or do something…they grab my hand and pull me to where they need to go."

"I say, 'Elizabeth, say cracker' or 'Emily, say marshmallow.' But I just keep saying it like that and they learn how to say it."

"…if they want to sit down and there's nothing there, sometimes they come and get you and they make you sit and they sit in your lap. So don't get really mad at that, that's just natural."

You've got to be pretty understanding to be willing to serve as an impromptu folding chair for your sisters. We interviewed Alex's mom, too. So we could at least partly see where he got his great attitude. After these interviews, we could almost hear mom's voice gently counseling, "That's just natural."

Make no mistake, not every child we interviewed was as patient as Alex, but they all had their strengths, and many had adapted to meet their siblings' needs.

Here's what Jacqueline said about learning to deal with her brother's meltdowns:

"Actually, nothing helps unless I do something funny. Sometimes I do funny faces or sometimes I just act silly, like run around the house…and he laughs."

DeP, whose brother is very high functioning and is "better at math than my mom and knows more about chemistry than my dad" had another approach:

"When he tries to take it out on me, my mom steps in. Then my dog comes in and she has this cute little face. She helps out my brother a lot. Then I just pick her up and give her to Cass. And he just holds her."

Other kids help their siblings communicate, Like Elianah:

"When he says something and the person that he's talking to doesn't understand him, I can understand him so I tell the person that Jaeden's talking to what he's saying."

Or Jonathan:

"I speak sign language to Kevin because that's the easiest way to communicate with him."

DeP also was one of the kids who explained how their relationships had improved, "I get along with him a lot better than I used to when I was about six or seven. We used to fight a lot back then, but now, we help each other out and we're pretty much tight brothers."

It was also great to hear kids bragging about their siblings, like Briceño, whose family discovered that his younger brother, who couldn't speak, had suddenly begun using one of his toys as a writing tool.

"Recinto's strengths – he's really good – at his last birthday there was just a big explosion. He loves to write letters on the little Magna Doodle thing and he's really good at that."

During our interviews, we found out a lot about how siblings learned to get along with their brothers and sisters and what parents tried that worked and didn't work. We heard about a range of issues, including kids often feeling that their siblings on the spectrum got more attention from mom and dad.

One quick insight. The families that seemed to be dealing best with autism or Asperger Syndrome made an effort to communicate early and often. It turns out many parents tend to think their kids know more about these conditions than they actually do. You might want to test this with your own kids. Sit down with them and talk. Explain why you're doing what you're doing. Ask them how they feel about things. You may get some input you can use to make things better in your family.

Well, I'm going back to editing videos. I may share more input from the interviews in the next few weeks. This project is sort of my world right now.

With all the help kids need from their parents understanding autism or Asperger Syndrome, you can't help but be impressed with some of the insights they come up with on their own. Like Jacqueline, explaining her brother's lack of speech skills:

"He doesn't really know how to talk that much, but I'm sure he's saying something in his mind."

Wow.

###

67 GIVING SIBLINGS THEIR DUE

Who do you love more, your child who has a condition such as Asperger Syndrome or autism -- or your child who doesn't? Dumb question? It may not seem so dumb to a child who sees his or her parents devoting large amounts of time to a brother or sister with special needs.

If you sometimes find that you're so focused on helping one child that your other children feel neglected or resentful, you're not alone. Let me share some suggestions I've gathered from families in this situation about improving understanding and cooperation.

1. Talk with siblings early and often about a special needs child's condition. Share appropriate information and explain what you're doing to help that child and why it's important. It's easy to assume that typically developing kids know more than they do about a sibling's special needs.
2. Listen to your children. If they have complaints or concerns, hear them out and show that you're seriously considering what they say before you reply. If they have reasonable concerns, act on them. If their concerns aren't reasonable, be patient and reassuring when you offer explanations. Consider holding both regular family meetings and individual conversations with each child.
3. Think of your child with special needs as a child first and a patient second. This helps him put his challenges in perspective, and helps you realistically balance his requirements with the needs of your other children.
4. Spend some regular one-on-one time with each child in your family doing something he or she enjoys. Even if one child's condition requires more of your time than another's, showing each child that he's special to you can go a long way toward gaining his understanding.

5. Pour on the praise when one child helps another. Making a child feel good about helping can encourage a behavior to become a habit.
6. Give each of your children the freedom to develop their individual identities and pursue their own interests. It's counterproductive to make siblings feel guilty when they want to do something by themselves at home or to spend some time alone with friends.
7. Find ways to give all your children roles in any therapies you do at home. If you can make therapy time fun, even better.
8. Seek out practical ways to include your special needs child in family activities, but don't get trapped into believing you have to include every child in every activity. If a special needs child can't sit quietly through a sibling's piano recital, find a trusted sitter so the rest of the family can attend. A mother I spoke with recently talked about getting a sitter for her son who has autism so that she, her husband and two neurotypical sons could occasionally eat out in a restaurant. This is a very caring family whose two older sons actively find things to do with their autistic younger brother. They've found a balance that's healthy for everyone.
9. Seek out appropriate support groups. A support group focused on your child's condition can offer information and camaraderie. A sibling support group can offer your neurotypical children the chance to interact with kids who understand their situation in ways other peers can't.
10. If you've got serious sibling issues, individual or family counseling may offer solutions you might not think of on your own.

Making sure all your children feel loved and appreciated encourages your family to work as a team to support each other. And a team can accomplish more than one person. So, if caring for your special needs child seems to monopolize your time, consider that finding more ways to show your other children that they're important could help ease the demands on you and improve the quality of life for every member of your family.

That's the kind of win-win scenario we're all looking for.

###

Dan Coulter

LIVING AS ADULTS

68 ADULT ASPERGER TACTICS FOR PARENTS

Does your child with Asperger Syndrome sometimes resist your guidance?

As the parents of an adult son with Asperger Syndrome, my wife and I have found that as a child gets older and feels the need to assert his or her independence, it may be harder and harder to take advice from mom or dad.

This is not necessarily a bad thing. It's important for our children to learn to solve their own problems. Especially as they become our adult children.

Still, it's tough to see the effectiveness of, "Because I said so," recede into the distance.

If we see a continuing need to be involved in our children's lives as they grow into adults, we need to acknowledge that they are becoming adults, and find appropriate ways to influence their decisions.

This can be a challenge.

People with Asperger Syndrome often have trouble with subtle distinctions. They may think, "Adults are independent. Being independent means making my own decisions. If I take my parents' advice, I'm not acting like an adult."

So, what do we do when we want to respect our children's quest for independence and still help them over or around a metaphorical brick wall?

The answer may lie in something I was told in military history class as a college ROTC cadet. The class was taught by a captain with a true Army man's loyalty and belief that his branch of the service was vastly superior to any other. One day in class, he was having fun at the expense of the Marines.

"In the Army, we believe in using strategy and tactics to capture an objective," he grinned. "But the Marines, the Marines have another approach, which can best be summed up as, 'Hey, diddle, diddle, straight up the middle, and the hell with everything else!'."

Of course, there were no Marines present. Had a Marine been present, I suspect we would have been treated to an enthusiastic corps-a-corps as to the accuracy of the captain's characterization. Not to mention speculations about the captain's parentage back through several generations.

But even assuming the captain's statement represented slander to the Marine Corps, the point is that the best tactic to use in providing counsel to your adult (or near adult) son or daughter may not be the direct approach.

Our 25 year-old son, Drew, was diagnosed with AS when he was 14. He has a B.A. in creative writing, but has gone back to school to complete a two-year college program in accounting. He hopes what he learns about accounting will help him land a full-time job. He's living at home and working part-time at our public library.

While he's done well in his accounting classes, Drew recently had difficulties with some long-term assignments for a complicated auditing course. He was frustrated and his mother and I were concerned. Drew made it clear that he wanted to prove he could handle this without his parents' help.

The solution involved my wife engaging the assistance of Drew's job coach. The coach met with Drew to work out a new plan, including studying in the library away from distractions. They came up with a schedule for completing parts of the assignments. This schedule included, if necessary, approaching the course's professor before the projects were due, to request additional time.

On his own, Drew enlisted a fellow student to explain some of the difficult concepts involved and started breaking down the obstacles that had caused his frustration. His mother and I were relieved. We were also impressed with Drew's initiative in seeking another student's help.

As parents of children with Asperger Syndrome, many of us get used to constantly having our hands on the safety net. We spend a lot of time wondering when to deploy it and when to whip it behind our backs and say, "What net?"

But if we can gradually forgo the direct approach and guide our children to find the help they need, even if it's not from us, we may just reach the Holy Grail point for parents. That's the point where our children are competent and confident enough to ask our advice because they value it, and not because they're afraid they can't succeed without it.

###

69 FUTURE PREPPING YOUR CHILD

Live in the moment. Prepare for the future.

Two good pieces of advice. Success and happiness require a bit of both.

Balancing the present and future is hard enough for parents, but it can be even harder for our children who have Asperger Syndrome or similar conditions. Many are firmly anchored in the "live in the moment" camp. But ready or not, the future is coming.

I got to thinking about this when my wife, Julie, told me about her day at a high school college fair. She stood at table among a roomful of other representatives ready to explain the virtues of her alma mater to students. After each discussion, the students were supposed to get the representative's signature on a card. I suppose this was to ensure that students didn't just use the event as an excuse to cut class.

Some students in the room were interested and engaged the college reps with questions about the curriculums and campuses and their futures. Others spent their time hanging around talking with their friends and pretty much ignoring the representatives. Except to occasionally dart to a table, extend an arm and ask, "Would you sign my card?"

Interested in the future vs. living in the moment. In an increasingly tough, global job market, who's on track for a happy, successful life?

But preparing for the future doesn't mean you can't enjoy yourself now.

The magic formula is merging the two concepts to get our children so fired up about a subject that they use it to shape their futures. Many of our offspring have a head start. I can't even count the children on the autism spectrum I've met who are passionate about a special interest.

Sure, I hear you say, but how do I convert my son's obsession with Japanese Anime or my daughter's passion about weather into a career?

First, do some research about your son or daughter's interest. Contact people in a related business and find out what jobs exist in that field. Then, take your child to meet some of those people. You don't have to limit your aspirations to an existing job. Assess your child's skills and ask the people you're meeting with if an employer might craft a new job around those skills.

Your weather-obsessed child may not be cut out to be an on-camera weather reporter, but might excel at building the computer models used in forecasting. If the skills your child has -- and wants to attain -- have value, you've got a shot. (If your child doesn't display a particular interest, perhaps your school could administer an aptitude test that could help you get the ball rolling.)

Your local community college also could be of help. Many have career programs and contacts with businesses you could use as resources. Or you could get in touch with your local chamber of commerce. Arranging a visit with a local artist or weather reporter could have a tremendous impact on even a young child. Set up these meetings with as many different people as possible. Discovering what your child doesn't want to do can be just as important as finding what he does. Remember, you're not working to absolutely determine your child's path. You're exposing him to possibilities and seeing what catches his imagination.

My son, Drew, has Asperger Syndrome. His special interests have changed over the years. When he was little, he was enthralled by Star Wars and Greek mythology. Later, he became fascinated with Japanese anime. But he's also interested in math and loves working with spreadsheets. At this point, he's hedging his bets, getting training in accounting so he can support himself while he finishes writing a book.

After getting a B.A. in creative writing, Drew went back to college for an accounting degree after we introduced him to an accountant and let him see what a job in that field would be like. And after he took a basic online accounting course to make doubly sure.

Business people often appreciate others who take the initiative. You may be surprised at the number of people who would be willing to talk with a student about their jobs. Especially if the student is excited about the visit. Some of these visits could even result in a part-time job or internship where your child can learn important job-related social skills. Unemployment is especially high among people with Asperger Syndrome, not because they don't have the skills to do a job, but because they have difficulty interacting with supervisors and co-workers. Outstanding job skills and a base level of social skills can be a winning combination for someone with Asperger Syndrome.

A part-time job in high school can help your child learn crucial workplace lessons that could make the difference in keeping a full time job later on. If it's too much to deal with a job after school hours, consider a summer job. But try as hard as you can to find something related to your child's interests.

Consider how your child reacts when asked to do something that doesn't appeal to him. Compare that to how animated he can be when urging you to let him do something he loves. I just know that when my son is not interested in something, working on it can be like a long hike in ill-fitting boots. When he is interested, he's winged Mercury.

Here's hoping you can link your child's passion to a career that makes preparing for the future one of the most fun things he can do with his moments.

He might just land a job ahead of the typically developing kids who spend their living-in-the-moment time hanging out instead of talking to representatives at a college fair.

Now wouldn't that be something?

70 PREPARING FOR A CAR ACCIDENT

I learned the value of the motto "Be Prepared" when I was a Boy Scout.

While you can't prepare for everything, you can anticipate likely events and plan for them, such as being in a car accident.

Car accidents are a concern for parents of children with Asperger Syndrome.

My wife and I frequently get asked by parents if our 24 year old son, Drew, who has Asperger Syndrome, drives. Yes. And he's a careful driver. So careful that he once spent a second too long looking down to make sure he was doing exactly the speed limit, and couldn't stop in time when the driver in front of him slammed on her brakes. There was bumper damage on each car, but no one was hurt. Since then, Drew has adapted his glance-down time.

Recently, Drew has been involved with two other accidents that were not his fault. Both were minor and no one was hurt. His first two "accident experiences" helped him learn the procedure for dealing with such situations. He was a lot more calm and confident dealing with the third incident.

Anyone can be shaken by a car accident, even a minor fender-bender. For some people, the aftermath of dealing with the other driver, witnesses and the police may seem more overwhelming than the collision.

After Drew's first fender-bender, I customized a "post accident checklist" and put copies in our family cars. I recommend everyone keep such a checklist, and go over what to do in case of an accident with every driver in the family.

Statistics tell us that even careful drivers risk having an accident sooner or later. Some accidents are unavoidable. Drew had one driver scrape his back bumper while he was stopped at a traffic light, and another suddenly pull into his path from a driveway.

Picture how each driver in your family would be likely to respond after an accident. Wouldn't it give you more peace of mind to provide them with some written instructions and maybe hold a practice session walking through what to do? You might even arrange for a police officer to talk with your son or daughter and explain what to expect.

Your car insurance agent can probably supply you with a "If You Have An Accident" checklist that you can personalize based on your family members' needs. Many insurance companies post such checklists on their websites.

At the end of this article, I've included a simple version of the accident checklist we keep in our cars, minus our personal information. This works for us. You need to determine what will work for you, based on your situation and your state and local laws. I'd recommend filling in your personal information beforehand and printing several copies. Also, you might want to put the documents in a three ring binder or on a clipboard so the driver has a portable writing surface -- and attach a pen.

I was able to be on the scene quickly after the most recent incident, where the car pulled out in front of Drew. While I was initially relieved to learn that no one was hurt, I felt a second wave of relief to see Drew dealing calmly and confidently with the other driver and the police.

This is the way you want your family member to be able to deal with this situation. Trust me.

###

The following pages contain a checklist you can copy and put in your car in case of an accident. Fill out any information you can in advance. Also, you may wish to attach these sheets to a clipboard and tie a pen to the clipboard with a string. That way you'll have a surface to write on and something to write with in those difficult moments right after an accident.

WHAT TO DO AFTER A CAR ACCIDENT

1 __ IF ANYONE IS SERIOUSLY HURT, CALL 911 AND SUMMON HELP.

2 __ CALL YOUR PARENTS.

Home: _____

Work: _____

Dad cell: _____

Mom Cell _____

3 __ CALL THE POLICE. If there is damage to the cars involved, call and report the accident to the police. Be ready to tell the police where you are. Look on a nearby building for a street address or look for the names of the two streets at a nearby intersection. Stay at the accident scene until the police arrive.

Police Phone Number: _____

4 ___ EXCHANGE INFORMATION WITH THE OTHER DRIVER OR DRIVERS INVOLVED.

(See attached sheets).

A. SHARE WRITTEN INFORMATION: Give him or her your name, address, phone number, car license number, car registration number, insurance company name and insurance policy number; and get the same information from him or her. It's best to have your information printed out and ready beforehand.

B. DON'T COMMENT: Do not tell the other driver if you think the accident was your fault or his fault.

C. DON'T ARGUE: If the other driver is uncooperative or attempts to argue with you, don't argue, just write down the license number of his car and wait for the police.

5 ___ COOPERATE WITH THE POLICE.

Stay calm. When the police arrive, follow their directions and answer their questions. Have your driver's license and registration ready for them.

When they ask, describe what happened briefly and clearly. Don't talk about things not directly connected to the accident. The police officer should give you a copy of his preliminary report, with the other driver's contact and insurance information, before the officer leaves the scene.

4 __ IF YOU CAN'T REACH YOUR PARENTS, CALL YOUR INSURANCE COMPANY. IF YOU REACHED YOUR PARENTS, CALL YOUR INSURANCE COMPANY AFTER YOU'VE TALKED WITH YOUR PARENTS.

Insurance Company Name _____

Insurance Policy Number: _____

Business Hours Phone: _____

After Business Hours Phone: _____

6 __ NOTE: Car registration and insurance card information are in an envelope in the car's glove compartment.

****

INFORMATION TO COLLECT FOR YOURSELF (Use more than one form if multiple other vehicles were involved.)

Other driver's information:

Name: _____

Address: _____

City: _____ State: _____ Zip Code: _____

Phone # s:

_____

Vehicle license #: _____

Vehicle registration #: _____

Make, model and year of other vehicle: _____

Insurance company name: _____

Insurance policy #: _____

Time of accident: _____

Date of accident: _____

Location of accident: (Near corner of two streets? Address of nearby building?)

_____

_____

_____

Describe damage to each car:

_____

_____

_____

_____

Names and phone numbers of witnesses, if any:

_____

_____

INFORMATION TO GIVE OTHER DRIVER

Your Name: _____

Your Address: _____

Your Phone Number: _____

Your car's year, make, model, car license number:

_____

Your car's registration number: _____

Your Insurance information:

Insurance Company Name: _____

Policy # _____

Phone: _____

ABOUT THE AUTHOR

Dan Coulter had no clue that he had Asperger Syndrome for most of his life. As a child, he was a bundle of contradictions. He was naïve, very literal and could miss implied meanings. He could get overwhelmed and find himself unable to speak. He had trouble gauging what other people were thinking -- and knowing the right thing to say in social situations. He had difficulty remembering people's names. He had a rigid adherence to rules and what was right and wrong.

At the same time, Dan was a voracious reader and gained a lot of knowledge early. He could remember some things in extraordinary detail. He did well in school and had a talent for writing and speaking. He had a knack for pointing out the humor in situations. He could see problems from different perspectives and sometimes solve them in innovative ways.

During high school, Dan learned to temper a tendency to talk a lot and worked on his listening skills.

At the University of Missouri at Columbia, Dan was named a University Scholar, graduated with honors and was elected to Phi Beta Kappa.

In his career, among other jobs, Dan has been a radio disk jockey, a television weatherman, a television writer/producer/director for AT&T, a national media spokesperson for AT&T, a media relations director for Bell Labs and a vice president of communications for telecom company Global Crossing.

After his son, Drew, was diagnosed with Asperger Syndrome, Dan started producing videos about the condition with his wife, Julie. Dan left corporate life to make educational videos full time in 2003. In 2004, Dan began writing and distributing articles about Asperger Syndrome which were posted on support group websites, printed in newsletters, and shared through Asperger and autism-related email distribution lists.

In 2009, Dan was diagnosed with Asperger Syndrome and began including the insights from the diagnosis in his videos, writings, and speaking engagements.

Dan and Julie now live in Winston-Salem, North Carolina, where Dan works compulsively at a job he loves, takes daily walks, and seriously considers getting a dog. Julie thinks a dog would help Dan mellow out.

We'll see.

Watch for Volume 2 of Dan Coulter's collected articles.

DVDS PRODUCED BY COULTER VIDEO

MANNERS FOR THE REAL WORLD - Basic Social Skills
Clear descriptions and demonstrations that help children and teenagers master common social skills.

ASPERGER SYNDROME AT WORK A guide to getting and keeping a job for people with Asperger Syndrome.

ASPERGER SYNDROME: Transition To College and Work How to search for and apply to the right college, how to access special needs services in college and how to prepare in high school for success in college. A separate section discusses developing skills for the workplace.

ASPERGER SYNDROME: Success In The Mainstream Classroom Includes interviews with parents, regular and special education teachers, a psychologist, an instructional aide and a social worker/case manager giving practical advice from their experience successfully integrating children with Asperger Syndrome into classrooms.

INTRICATE MINDS: Understanding Classmates with Asperger Syndrome Candid interviews with teenagers designed to promote positive interactions between classmates and reduce isolation, harassment and bullying. For middle school and high school.

INTRICATE MINDS II: Understanding Elementary School Classmates With Asperger Syndrome This video features interviews with elementary school students explaining how Asperger Syndrome affects them and describing their challenges and strengths. Designed to promote positive interactions between elementary school classmates.

INTRICATE MINDS III: Understanding Elementary School Classmates Who Think Differently This video is another version of Intricate Minds II that doesn't focus on a single diagnosis. With modified narration and additional interviews, it promotes understanding for children with a range of conditions including Asperger Syndrome, Higher Functioning Autism, Pervasive Developmental Delay, Semantic-Pragmatic Disorder and others.

ASPERGER SYNDROME FOR DADS: Becoming An Even Better Father To Your Child With AS Ten secrets parents can use to help a child with AS reach his full potential and have fun along the way.

UNDERSTANDING BROTHERS AND SISTERS with ASPERGER SYNDROME Helps siblings of different ages understand and accept brothers and sisters with Asperger Syndrome.

UNDERSTANDING BROTHERS AND SISTERS on the AUTISM SPECTRUM Helps siblings of different ages understand and accept brothers and sisters with a range of autism spectrum behaviors.

(The two sibling videos are similar in approach but different in content. One features families dealing with Asperger Syndrome, the other with autism.)

You can find more information at www.coultervideo.com.

Life in the Asperger Lane